The Woman's Migraine Toolkit

Managing Your Headaches from Puberty to Menopause

Dawn A. Marcus, MD
Professor, Department of Anesthesiology
University of Pittsburgh
Pittsburgh, Pennsylvania

Philip A. Bain, MD
Department of Internal Medicine
Dean Health System
Madison, Wisconsin

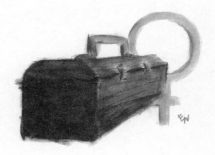

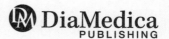
DiaMedica
PUBLISHING

DiaMedica Publishing, 150 East 61st Street, New York, NY 10065

Visit our website at www.diamedicapub.com

Library of Congress Cataloging-in-Publication Data is available from the publisher.

DiaMedica titles are available for bulk purchase, special promotions, and premiums. For more information please contact the publisher through the publisher's website: www.diamedicapub.com.

Disclaimer:
The content in this book is not intended as a substitute for medical or professional counseling and advice. The reader is encouraged to consult his or her physicians and therapists on all health matters, especially symptoms that may require professional diagnosis and/or medical attention.

ISBN: 978-0-9823219-2-8

Book and cover design by Gopa & Ted2
Illustrations by Ian S. Klipa
Design by TypeWriting
Editing by Jessica Bryan, Joann Woy

Contents

Praise for *The Woman's Migraine Toolkit*

". . . (The book) is well laid out and organized into sections that make it easy to read, whether you're reading it straight through or looking for specific information. The illustrations add to the information without distracting from it. A wide range of possible treatments are discussed . . . The information about medications is supplemented with helpful charts for comparison and quick reference . . . packed with valuable information that's presented in a way that's easy to refer to again later. With bulleted lists, charts, and relevant illustrations, this is one of the best presentations of large amounts of information you can find in print."

—Teri Robert, Patient Advocate and Author,
Living Well with Migraine Disease and Headache

". . . a bedrock foundation of essential practical information that can be built upon. . . I spend a great deal of time educating my patients about their condition and what it will take to control the chaos that has become their migraines. At the end of the day there is never enough time in the day to do it all by yourself. *The Woman's Migraine Toolkit* is a perfect partner to pick up where my appointments leave off. . ."

—Michael Ready, MD, Director, Headache Clinic,
Scott and White Memorial Hospital, Temple, Texas

". . . a comprehensive yet clear and readable review of migraine that targets issues of particular importance to women. . . It contains practical advice and action steps that you can take on your own, advice on how to talk with your health care provider about your migraine, and questionnaires and logs that you can complete and share with your health care provider."

—Dawn Buse, M.D. Department of Neurology,
Albert Einstein College of Medicine, Bronx, New York,
and Director of Behavioral Medicine, Montefiore Headache Center

" . . . a useful toolkit for the woman who wishes not only to understand her migraines, but to be an active participant in her treatment. Clearly organized into sections that speak directly to its audience . . . each generously endowed with charts and illustrations . . . chock full of calendars, diets, exercises, and websites. It answers common questions, addresses pharmacologic and non-pharmacologic approaches to treatment, and even offers advice on how to be more effective in communicating with your physician."

Anne H. Calhoun, M.D., Carolina Headache Institute,
Chapel Hill

" . . . highly recommended for its clarity, to-the-point simplicity, yet depth of information. (The book) begins with a complete explanation of the biology and causes of migraine it terms that a patient can relate to. It clearly summarizes what happens to women as they go through their hormonal changes from young girls to postmenopausal adults, accurately depicts the many phases and problems of migraine, and an exhaustive body of information on all types of therapy . . . It really *is* a toolkit, explaining best treatments of all aspects of your headache and all points in your life. It closes with helpful hints on talking to your doctor and an excellent and complete resource guide. I will recommend it often to my patients."

—Alan M. Rapoport, M.D., Clinical Professor of Neurology, UCLA;
Founder and Director-Emeritus,
The New England Center for Headache

". . . holds a wealth of information for understanding as well as managing migraine. As the title indicates, the book is directed toward the woman headache sufferer, with chapters on treating migraine during menses, pregnancy, and menopause. The chapter on hormones was my personal favorite; I found it comprehensive yet cogent . . . I tried to read the book from a patient's rather than a physician's perspective, and found the explanations to be logical and well-structured, and the writing style fluid. The shaded boxes highlighting treatment tips as well as important information and summaries, add to the readability . . . an outstanding resource for the well-educated reader, including health professionals who treat migraine."

—Gretchen Tietjen, MD, Professor and Chair of Neurology,
Director of the UTMC Headache Treatment
and Research Center, University of Toledo

" . . . a must read for all women with migraines. This book explains in an easy to read and easy to understand format what causes migraines, why women are more likely to get migraines, and how hormonal changes influence migraines. More importantly, this book empowers women with the knowledge of what they can do to manage their migraines. How to use relaxation techniques, biofeedback, and stretching exercises are explained with easy step-by-step instructions and illustrations. . . Included is a thorough discussion of which medications are safe during pregnancy, breastfeeding, and menopause. This is a well-written, comprehensive guide that I will highly recommend to all my migraine patients. As a gynecologist who treats many female migraine patients, this is the book I have been waiting for. *The Woman's Migraine Toolkit* will enable women to take control of their migraine management and work with their physicians to set up a treatment plan that works for them. Knowledge is Power."

—Debra L. Hill-Busselle M.D., FACOG, Gynecologist and Women's
Healthcare Specialist, Bozeman, MT

"If any of you are migraine sufferers or live with someone who gets them, please get this book. It is very hard for people who do not get migraines to understand how debilitating they can be for those who do and this book does a wonderful job of explaining what it is we experience. . . Please, please, please, if you love someone who has migraines (including yourself) get this book so you can help them help themselves to handle and even perhaps prevent these debilitating headaches. Life is too short to spend it in pain when it isn't necessary.

—The 1000 Book List

". . . very informative . . . a good, helpful book for women who suffer from migraines."

—Amazon Early Reviewer

"On the whole I liked this book. It's accessible, friendly, and reassuring. A lot of the advice it offers is immediately useful, both in terms of understanding the migraine experience and managing it. It includes things like stretches and exercises, suggestions for communicating with health-care providers, discussions of various medications and alternative medicine approaches, and the genetics of migraine susceptibility . . ."

—Amazon Earlier Reviewer

" . . . great information on relaxation stretches, drug and herbal treatments, diet triggers—all sorts of things to help someone cope with migraines. It discusses current medical models of migraines . . . It also has a wonderful section I wish I had read years ago on preparing for a medical appointment. I think the information there would be incredibly useful and empowering in that setting . . . I highly recommend this book, especially for someone newly diagnosed . . ."

—Amazon Early Reviewer

The subtitle of this book is "Managing Your Headaches from Puberty to Menopause," and that pretty much covers the book. I consider myself pretty knowledgeable about migraines. I've suffered from them since I was 13, and witnessed my mother coping with them to the point of hospitalization. From the very beginning of this book, though, I learned new things—such as that I've been medicating myself at the wrong stage of the cycle, which is why drugs often do very little to help with the pain . . . I appreciated the book's approach, which is easy to understand for laymen but not dumbed down, either. Chapters outline possible treatments, ranging from massage techniques to prescriptions to natural remedies . . . This is one I'll be keeping on my shelf—that is, after I let my mom borrow it.

—LibraryThing Reviewer

Preface

Awoman's life is a time of exciting changes, as the early curves of puberty blossom into womanhood, bringing the possibilities of motherhood. Today, women's lives are open to a full range of possible roles—daughter, friend, mother, spouse, and professional. In many ways, women have never had as many choices as they have today. For many women, however, their options become limited from disabling and recurring migraines.

If you have migraines, you're not alone. Migraine affects 18 percent of adult women—one in six women suffer from these distressing headaches. Migraines are much more than "just a headache." They can affect your whole life—resulting in countless days of missed work and school, reduced productivity, and limits on your participation in family activities and social events. To some women, migraine may feel like a curse. Migraine sufferers often feel hopeless and helpless, destined to suffer in silence. They may have seen healthcare providers in the past but stopped seeing them, either because of ineffective treatment or a perceived lack of communication. Many are discouraged and frustrated. Twenty years ago, suffering and despair was the norm.

The good news is that we now have a much better understanding about what causes migraines and how to get them under control. Many advances in diagnosis and treatment have been made in recent years, giving new hope to women suffering from these disabling headaches. Women are taking control of their headaches by seeking out those providers who are interested in treating headache, learning all they can about migraines, and taking an active role in caring for patients. Expectations for better headache management have increased, and rightfully so.

The Woman's Migraine Toolkit provides the practical headache information you need to control your migraine headaches. We discuss migraines from childhood through menopause, explaining how each hormonal milestone affects headache patterns and how to best monitor, treat, and control them. You'll probably find that you'll need different treatments when you're an adult, compared to when you were a child. During some life stages—such as when you're pregnant—you'll need treatment options that are safest for you and your baby.

A wide range of effective therapeutic options is available for treating migraine symptoms and preventing future headaches from occurring. *The Woman's Migraine Toolkit* will show you when you should use different therapies and which treatments work better during the different stages of your life. In addition to over-the-counter and prescription medications, effective non-drug treatments and nutritional supplements are available. Throughout this book, you'll find practical instructions about all types of treatments, as well as tools to help monitor your headaches and decide if the treatment you're using is the best one for you.

One unique feature of the book is a section on how to talk to your doctor about your headaches, and how to make the most of your office visits. In this section, you'll learn how to overcome common barriers to effective communication with your healthcare provider, to help make sure you're both "on the same page" with your headache treatment. The Resource Guide lists a wide range of reliable sources for all aspects of headache care.

We believe migraine sufferers need more than just a medication prescription—they need a comprehensive, holistic approach to headache management that addresses diet, sleep patterns, exercise habits, mood, and social concerns, in addition to drug therapy. Your migraine treatment strategy must consider all aspects of your life, as well as what your headaches are like and what type of treatments best meet your lifestyle needs. The more treatment options you learn about, the better chance you'll have for finding the treatment approach that works best for you.

In *The Woman's Migraine Toolkit*, you'll notice that we often use the words "migraine" and "headache" interchangeably. We do this because many women with recurring headaches don't recognize that their attacks—especially milder attacks—are migraine. We often hear patients talk about their "migraines" and their "regular headaches." Much of the time, those "regular headaches" are just milder forms of migraine. Some women don't realize their attacks can be migraine unless they vomit during an episode. Other women will say, "I don't get migraines like my mom or sister—mine are just normal headaches," not realizing that migraine attacks can have different features in different women.

It's important to understand when your episodes are migraine for several reasons. First, migraine is much more than just a headache. In this book, you'll read about the wide range of symptoms women can experience with migraine. And, in some cases, a migraine attack can occur where the headache is a very mild symptom or there's no headache at all. Second, migraine is not just a reaction to stress—it's a real biological condition. And third, there are many effective treatments for migraine. You don't need to suffer or feel like "it's just a headache."

You don't have to let your migraines control your life—take charge by learning what causes migraines, how to evaluate your headaches, how to effectively communicate with your healthcare provider so that you can work as a team to get your headaches under better control. *The Woman's Migraine Toolkit* contains instructions and resources to take you from your first headaches in puberty through your adult years. Learn how to control your migraine symptoms and reclaim your life!

Dawn A. Marcus, MD
Pittsburgh, Pennsylvania

Philip A. Bain, MD
Madison, Wisconsin

Acknowledgments

Thanks to Ian Klipa for adding eye-catching art to this book and to Cheryl Noethiger, Diana Hare, and Anita Mohan for providing their images to show migraines and migraine treatments.

An Overview of Migraine

What Are Migraines? Why Me?

Do you ever feel like no one really understands what your headaches are like? Do you ever wonder if you're the only one who gets migraine episodes like yours? You should know that migraine is actually very common. Nearly 30 million Americans suffer from migraine, making it one of the most frequent medical conditions. In fact, migraine is more common than asthma and diabetes combined. Migraine disproportionately affects women. Before puberty, boys and girls are equally likely to have migraine headaches. After puberty, girls have a much higher risk of getting migraines, and they continue to be more common in women throughout their lives.

UNDERSTANDING THE BIOLOGY OF MIGRAINE

What exactly is migraine? Migraine is nothing new. Historical documents show that people have had migraines for thousands of years. Writings from Babylon in 3000 BC and scrolls buried with Egyptian mummies about 1500 BC describe migraines. Hippocrates, the Father of Modern Medicine, also wrote extensive descriptions of migraine. Many experts believe that the visionary artwork produced by the medieval

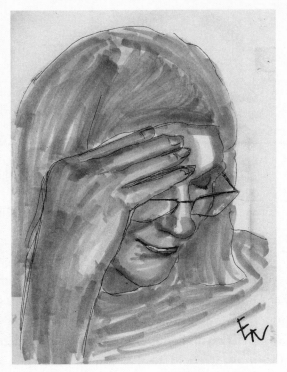

Women have been experiencing migraines—sick headaches with a common desire to shield the eyes from painful light—for 1000s of years.

nun Hildegard of Bingen included images attributable to migraine symptoms. When you get a migraine, you may experience the same distortions in vision that Hildegard showed in her art, including common migraine aura symptoms such as visual hallucinations of stars, zigzag lines, and blind spots.

Over time, medical research has learned more about the causes of migraine. This has resulted in a change in the language used to describe migraine. Older terms such as *vascular headache* (suggesting that the main problem in migraine involves blood vessels) and *sick headache* (referring to nausea and disability with migraines) have been replaced by the term *migraine*. The table below shows the current definition of migraine, according to the International Headache Society. These diagnostic criteria are used most commonly in headache research. A more

INTERNATIONAL HEADACHE SOCIETY DEFINITION OF MIGRAINE	
General description	Chronic, disabling, recurring, intermittent headache
Typical headache duration in adults	4 hours to 3 days
At least two of these four features	Pain is mainly on one side of the head Pain is throbbing or pulsing Pain is moderate or severe, limiting activities Doing regular activities (such as climbing stairs or bending forward) makes the pain worse
At least one of these two features	Sensitivity to lights and noises Nausea or vomiting
Temporary aura symptoms occur before or with migraine in about one in five migraine sufferers	Most commonly visual hallucinations, such as seeing colored balls, sparkling lights, zigzag lines, or blind spots

practical definition, and one that many doctors use, is that *migraine is a very common, controllable group of symptoms, in addition to headache, that is often inherited and clearly has a biological basis.*

Let's break down the individual components of this definition of migraine. First, migraine is very common, affecting 12 percent of all adults—6 percent of men and 18 percent of women. That's one in every six women! These figures are remarkably consistent in countries around the world. That's a staggering figure. So,

One in six women suffer from migraines.

as you read this book, remember—*you are not alone*—many women just like you suffer from migraines.

Next, migraine is very controllable, although not curable. With a proper diagnosis and an effective headache treatment plan, the vast majority of migraine sufferers can lead normal, productive lives. An effective treatment strategy that involves lifestyle changes, non-drug treatments, and medications can dramatically reduce lost time from work and family activities, and significantly improve quality of life.

Migraine Is More Than Just a Headache

Migraine is more than just a headache. Migraine includes a constellation of pain and non-pain symptoms. Most migraine attacks can be divided into four phases:

- ► Prodrome
- ► Aura
- ► Headache symptoms (includes pain)
- ► Postdrome

You may experience all or only some of these phases with your migraines, and you may have different phases during different migraine episodes.

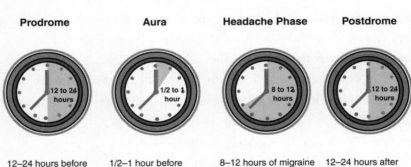

Prodrome	Aura	Headache Phase	Postdrome
12 to 24 hours	1/2 to 1 hour	8 to 12 hours	12 to 24 hours

12–24 hours before headache
- Irritability
- Neck pain
- Food cravings
- Yawning

1/2–1 hour before headache
- Affects 1 in 5 people with migraine
- Vision changes
- Numbness
- Weakness
- Dizziness
- Confusion

8–12 hours of migraine symptoms
- Throbbing headache
- Nausea
- Sensitivity to lights
- Sensitivity to noise
- Sensitivity to odors
- Disability or limited activities

12–24 hours after headache
- Hung-over feeling
- Fatigue
- Poor concentration

Phases of migraine.

The Prodrome Phase

The first phase of migraine, the *prodrome*, occurs in about one in three migraine sufferers. Although some people talk about the prodrome being distinct from and occurring before a migraine, many experts believe the prodrome is actually the first phase of an entire migraine episode. If you consistently experience prodrome symptoms before your headache phase, you can use this information to begin treating your migraine earlier. In some cases, treating the prodrome prevents the headache phase from developing.

One migraine sufferer in three has symptoms (called a prodrome) several hours to a day before the painful headache phase of migraine. Watch for any possible prodrome symptoms, so that you can start treatment earlier and possibly prevent the headache from occurring.

The prodrome typically begins about 12–24 hours before the headache phase. Some people have prodrome symptoms that last for 2 days before the headache phase. During this phase, you may experience a variety of non-specific symptoms:

- ▶ Changes in mood:
  - Irritability
  - Hyperactivity
  - Anxiety
  - Depression
- ▶ Digestive symptoms:
  - Food cravings (often carbohydrates and chocolate)
  - Diarrhea
  - Constipation
  - Loss of appetite
- ▶ Neck pain
- ▶ Neurologic symptoms:
  - Difficulty concentrating
  - Dizziness
  - Blurred vision

- Sensitivity to noises or lights
▶ Excessive yawning
▶ Frequent urination

In some cases, your friends and family may be helpful in identifying your prodrome symptoms. If they say they can tell that you're going to get a headache the next day, ask them how they know and keep track of the symptoms in a migraine diary. (See a sample headache diary later in the chapter.)

The Aura Phase

An *aura* is a temporary abnormality of nerve function that typically lasts for 5 minutes to an hour. Auras occur in about 10 to 20 percent of

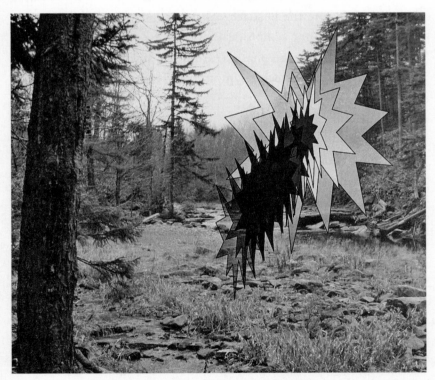

An aura often affects vision. You may develop colored, shimmery lines that travel across your vision. As the lines move across your sight, you may be left with a temporary blind spot.

people with migraine, or up to one in five migraine sufferers. The aura typically starts about one-half to one hour before the headache phase; however, auras can also occur after the headache phase has started.

Auras most commonly involve changes in vision, but many other nerve functions may be affected. Common aura symptoms include:

- ▶ Vision changes:
  - Flashing lights
  - Zigzag lines
  - Blurry vision
  - Blind spots or black holes
  - Distorted images
- ▶ Numbness on one side of the body
- ▶ Weakness on one side of the body
- ▶ Dizziness
- ▶ Confusion

One of the more interesting visual aura symptoms is a peculiar distortion of visual images called *metamorphopsia*, or change in the perception of size. During metamorphopsia, what migraine sufferers see is distorted, with some parts of objects appearing too big and others too small. Headache experts believe that Lewis Carroll must have been inspired by his own metamorphopsia when he wrote about Alice seeing things get bigger and smaller in *Through the Looking Glass*.

Interestingly, sometimes aura symptoms can occur without a headache. This is often seen in older people—especially after age 40. This is called *aura without migraine*, or *acephalgic* migraine. Auras can be frightening because they are so unusual. Many people fear they are having a stroke. *If there's a change in your aura or you develop a new aura, be sure to see your doctor.*

It is important to identify when an aura is part of the migraine pattern, because women who have auras are at slightly higher risk for strokes. The risk of having a stroke in people who don't get migraines

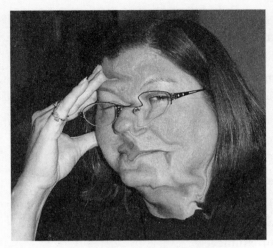

Images are often blurred and distorted during a migraine.

is about 19 strokes for every 100,000 people. The risk of stroke is nearly doubled in women who have migraine auras, to about 35 in 100,000 women. The good news is that the overall risk of getting a stroke is quite small, because you're doubling an already small number. Stroke risk is not significantly increased in women who have migraine without aura.

Women with a migraine aura have a slightly increased risk for stroke. So, if you get auras, make sure you stay heart-healthy to minimize your risk. Also, do not smoke and avoid estrogen-containing oral contraceptives, if at all possible.

A more important risk for women with aura is an increased stroke risk if they are *also* using oral contraceptives that contain estrogen. Stroke risk increases in women who have migraine with aura and also use estrogen-containing oral contraceptives to 75 strokes per 100,000. If you have aura, are a smoker, *and* use birth control pills, your risk increases even more, to over 100 strokes per 100,000.

If you have migraine with aura, you can reduce your stroke risk by:

▶ Keeping your weight in check
▶ Controlling your blood pressure

▶ Eating a low-fat diet and monitoring your blood lipid levels (cholesterol and triglycerides)
▶ Exercising regularly
▶ Avoiding smoking
▶ Consider using estrogen-containing oral contraceptives as a last resort, and only after thorough discussion with your healthcare professional

Remember, even though stroke risk increases in women with migraine with aura, the overall risk for stroke is relatively low and should not cause undue alarm. Migraine without aura is not associated with an increased risk of stroke.

Aura symptoms, like prodrome symptoms, can also serve as a warning that the headache phase of a migraine will soon begin. The aura phase can give you another chance to begin your migraine treatment early, thereby minimizing or avoiding the headache phase.

The Headache Phase

The headache phase can be subdivided into early headache, mid-headache, and late headache phases. Headaches often start out as mild during the early phase, build in intensity over the mid-headache phase, and then diminish during the late phase. Headaches may start on one side during the early headache phase and then spread to involve the entire head as severity intensifies during the mid-headache phase. In most people, the headache phase lasts about 8–24 hours in adults and 2–4 hours in children with migraine.

Although termed the *headache* phase, migraine sufferers usually also experience a variety of other unpleasant and disabling symptoms during this phase:

▶ Extreme sensitivity to noises, lights, and odors
▶ A strong desire to isolate oneself

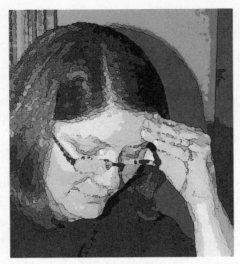

Migraines can affect all of the senses. Pain can sometimes be reduced by pressing on the temples during an attack.

▶ Nausea and vomiting
▶ Imbalance, including dizziness, unsteadiness, and room spinning

These symptoms can lead to significant disability during a migraine, causing you to leave work, find alternatives for childcare, and retreat to a quiet, dark room. Many people are entirely unable to function during a severe attack. An effective headache treatment strategy can significantly reduce the disability associated with the headache phase.

The headache phase *typically includes throbbing head pain, extreme sensitivity to noises, lights, and odors, and nausea.*

Treating during the early headache phase, while symptoms are less severe, can dramatically reduce symptom severity during the later stages of the headache phase and also reduce the duration of the headache phase. A good marker for determining when to treat is by monitoring your headache phase for the development of touch sensitivity, which is referred to as *cutaneous allodynia*. (*Cutaneous* means skin and *allodynia* means "different pain" or pain resulting from a normally non-painful action.) In this case, a gentle touch that would not normally be perceived as causing pain is felt as something painful. This is similar to sunburn—before the sunburn, touching your skin produces no pain. After a day in the scorching sun, that same gentle, light touch can feel very painful.

Monitor your headache phase for cutaneous allodynia (touch sensitivity). Try to treat your migraine before this begins for best results.

During a migraine, you may feel cutaneous allodynia in several ways:

▶ You may find it uncomfortable to wear jewelry or glasses.
▶ You may feel as if your "hair hurts."
▶ You may not want people to touch you.

Once you start to feel symptoms of touch sensitivity, typical migraine medications are usually much less effective compared with taking the same medication before the allodynia started. Many headache experts have coined the phrase "the race to allodynia" to emphasize that migraines should be treated before touch sensitivity occurs, in order to ensure better migraine relief success.

The Postdrome Phase

The fourth and final phase of migraine is the *postdrome* phase. Almost three of every four people who suffer from migraine experience a migraine postdrome. This phase starts after the symptoms during the headache phase have faded, and it typically lasts for several hours to 1 day.

The most commonly used description of the postdrome is "headache hangover." Migraine sufferers typically describe a variety of symptoms:

▶ Fatigue and a drained feeling
▶ Feeling washed out
▶ Feeling like being "in a fog"
▶ Difficulty concentrating
▶ Having low-grade pain or discomfort

A postdrome is the hung-over feeling, the so-called "migraine fog" that can linger for a day or so after the headache phase of migraine has resolved.

The postdrome can substantially extend the time of disability experienced with migraine. This is why people may need 12–24 or even up to 48 hours after a severe migraine to feel like they're "back to normal."

Putting the Migraine Phases Together

As you can see, a migraine isn't just a headache, but rather a wide range of unpleasant and often disabling symptoms. The time frame of a headache episode is quite variable. Features of an "average" migraine are shown on page 13. Monitoring the time to peak headache is a useful concept for migraine sufferers. Although the average time to the worst headache symptoms is 3 hours, some migraines peak within a few minutes or a couple of hours, while others may take a day or longer to reach maximum severity. If your migraines typically peak very quickly, you'll want to treat very early in your migraine episode. If you use medications, you may prefer to use those medications that get into the bloodstream more quickly than oral tablets, such as nasal sprays or injections.

Understanding the progression of your headache is important. Quickly peaking headaches or headaches that wake you may require non-pill approaches— including faster-acting options such as nasal sprays or injections.

Another important aspect of the concept of time to peak intensity is that some people wake up with a severe headache, and the usual oral medications don't work well. These are often the headaches that make them miss work or school, or that send them to the emergency room. The explanation for this is that, for some reason, the headache began during sleep and, by the time they woke up, they were already into the difficult-to-treat cutaneous allodynia phase. If this happens to you, you may not respond well to oral medications when you wake up with a migraine, and you may get better relief with non-oral forms of medications, such as nasal sprays or injections.

FEATURES OF THE AVERAGE MIGRAINE

▶ Half of all migraine sufferers have attacks beginning at varying times during the day:

- For one migraine sufferer in five, most migraines begin in the morning.
- For one migraine sufferer in seven, most migraines begin in the afternoon.

▶ The average duration of a migraine is 29 hours.

▶ The average time to peak headache (the worst symptoms) is 3 hours.

MIGRAINE IS OFTEN INHERITED

Why do I have migraines? Are they genetic? Did Mom give me her headaches, and will I give them to my children?

Like many health conditions, migraine is probably caused by a combination of genetic and environmental factors. Migraine tends to run in families, more often on the mother's side. Between half and two-thirds of people with migraine headaches have close relatives who also have them.

Studies of twins confirm that there is an important genetic component to migraines. A study of more than 8,000 adult twin pairs found that when one twin had migraines, an identical twin—who shares the same genetics—was over twice as likely to also have migraines, compared with a nonidentical twin, who has different genetics. This shows that about half the risk for migraine comes from your genes. The other half comes from environmental factors. In general, you have about a 50 percent chance of getting migraines if one of your parents has migraine, and a 75 percent chance if

A tendency for migraine is often inherited. When one twin has migraine, an identical twin is twice as likely to also have migraine.

A. When **both parents** have migraine, so will **three of every four of their children**

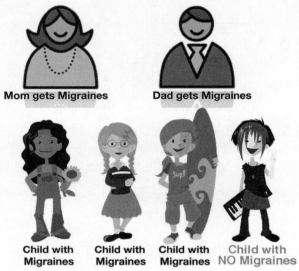

Mom gets Migraines   Dad gets Migraines

Child with   Child with   Child with   Child with
Migraines   Migraines   Migraines   NO Migraines

B. When **one parent** gets migraines, so will **half of their children**

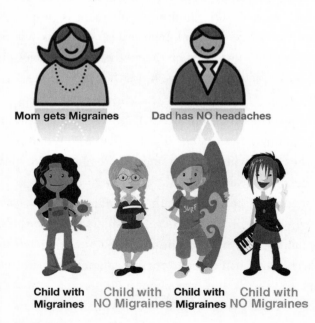

Mom gets Migraines   Dad has NO headaches

Child with   Child with   Child with   Child with
Migraines   NO Migraines   Migraines   NO Migraines

Migraines run in families.

both parents have migraine. Even if neither parent has migraine, you might still develop migraine, in which case you may pass the condition on to your children.

When one parent has migraine, the child will have a 50 percent chance of developing migraine. When both parents have migraine, the child's risk increases to 75 percent.

Despite extensive study, researchers have still not discovered "the migraine gene." While some rare forms of migraine involve alterations or *mutations* in one or just a few genes, the common variety of migraine probably involves multiple genes. Abnormalities in several individual genes have been linked to an increased risk for migraine, as shown in the table on page 16. Humans have 23 pairs of chromosomes, numbered 1 through 23. Chromosomes look like an "X" with short arms at the top and long arms at the bottom. The letter "p" in a chromosome's name refers to the short arms, and "q" refers to the long arms. Most studies have shown abnormalities on regions located on the short arms of chromosome 19 (or 19p) and the long arms of chromosome 1 (or 1q). The strongest links have been shown for chromosome abnormalities in patients with *familial hemiplegic* migraine, a rare form of migraine that causes headache with prolonged weakness or paralysis of half of the body, in conjunction with the migraine.

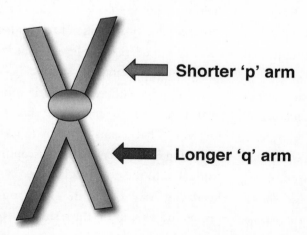

Shorter 'p' arm

Longer 'q' arm

Typical chromosome.

ABNORMALITIES IN SEVERAL GENES HAVE BEEN LINKED TO MIGRAINE

Type of migraine	Chromosome
Migraine with aura	4q24
	19p13
Migraine without aura	14q21.2-q22.3
Familial hemiplegic migraine*	19p13
	1q31
	1q23
	2q24

*This is a rare type of migraine that runs in families and causes a headache with marked weakness of one side of the body or paralysis.

Genetics Is Just One Factor

Inheriting a tendency for migraine means that your brain and nervous system are more prone to respond to exposure to certain headache triggers by getting a migraine; in other words, you have an increased vulnerability or susceptibility to migraine. This is where the concepts of *susceptibility* and *threshold* come in. People who are more susceptible to developing migraines will develop them in response to very low levels of a stimulus, whereas people who are not migraine-prone will not respond to the same level of stimulus. The term *threshold* refers to the level at which a stimulus will produce a reaction in specific individuals.

If you inherit an increased susceptibility to having migraine, you will be more prone to having headaches. But you may or may not develop migraines.

Migraine sufferers similarly inherit a lowered threshold or increased susceptibility to migraine. That means exposure to fewer triggers will bring on a headache in a susceptible person, compared to the non-headache prone person. A headache may occur in even non-headache prone individuals if they stay up too late at night, skip breakfast, have a very stressful day, *and* drink some red wine. For the headache-prone individual, exposure to just one of these potential triggers may result in a headache.

Migraine Clearly Has a Biological Basis

What happens during a migraine? Are migraines biological or just an emotional reaction?

Migraine is definitely a real, biological condition that is caused by chemical imbalances in the brain and nervous system.

Although stress is a common trigger for migraine, this does not mean migraine is an emotional or psychological disorder. Most real medical conditions get worse when we're under stress—stomach problems, chest pain, tremors, and even epilepsy. Stress doesn't *cause* any of these medical conditions—but it can make symptoms more apt to occur—just like migraines.

The threshold concept helps to clarify the role of stress and other triggers for headaches. When a person with a lowered threshold to headache comes in contact with a trigger, a series of events begins. Sometimes migraine triggers are obvious, like drinking red wine, having your menstrual period, or having a stressful day; other times, triggers are less clear and may be internal changes in the body of which we're unaware.

After the migraine process has been initiated, nerve cell activity in the back of the brain (the *occipital*, or *visual*, *cortex*) begins moving to the front to the brain. This wave of nerve activity is noted on both sides of the brain. The wave initially causes the nerve cells to be less active, and a wave of increased nerve activity follows. Because migraine activity often begins in the part of the brain affecting vision, many migraine sufferers experience visual changes during their attacks, such as migraine auras and blurred vision. An area of the brain called the *hypothalamus* is also activated. This causes the vague feelings of irritability, anxiety, hyperactivity, food crav-

> *Migraine is a threshold disorder. When the threshold is exceeded, a migraine occurs.*

ings, and increased urination that are reported as prodrome symptoms by some people with migraine.

As the nerves become activated, the ends of the nerves next to blood vessels in the scalp (outside the skull) release certain chemicals, such as *serotonin*, which cause the blood vessels to expand or dilate and become inflamed. These expanded blood vessels cause an increase in the blood flow around the brain. As a result, you may notice that the blood vessels at your temples increase in size and are tender. Other chemicals are also released from the nerve endings, leading to more dilated and inflamed blood vessels. These dilated, inflamed blood vessels further stimulate the nerve endings to release more chemicals, thereby amplifying the process.

The migraine process involves nerves, nerve endings, blood vessels, and various parts of the brain and brainstem.

Once nerve activation starts, nerves located in the brainstem begin to send migraine messages throughout the brain. Pain signals are transmitted to the muscles in the neck, which become stiff and painful. This causes the neck pain that is often seen during both the prodrome and headache phases of migraine. Pain signals also travel to the part of the brain sometimes referred to as the "nausea center," resulting in loss of

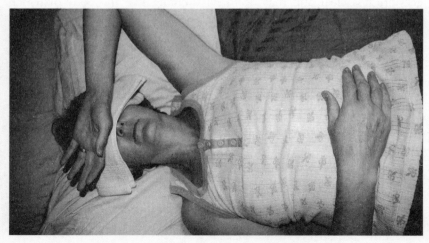

When a migraine becomes full blown, people often take to bed and get comfort by placing a cool cloth over their temple, forehead, or eyes.

appetite, nausea, and sometimes even vomiting. Pain messages also travel to pain centers in the brain, further amplifying the pain response. At this point, the process has cascaded out of control, resulting in what some people call a "full-blown" migraine.

Migraines used to be referred to as *vascular headaches* because scientists believed the entire process was primarily related to blood vessel changes. Over time—as more pieces of the migraine puzzle were discovered—the blood vessel theory was replaced by the neurovascular model described earlier. (*Neuro* means nerve and *vascular* means blood vessels.) The current theory of migraine recognizes the important interactions between nerves and blood vessels, which eventually result in the symptoms experienced as a migraine. The various migraine treatments that you will read about in this book work by affecting different aspects of the migraine mechanism. When you use a migraine treatment, you're targeting different biological abnormalities—not just covering up symptoms.

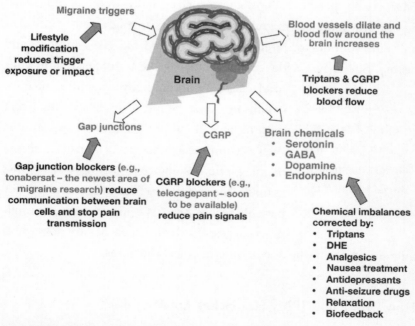

An overview of treatments you'll read about in later chapters, showing you which parts of the migraine pathway are affected by each treatment. Gap junction and CGRP blocker drugs are currently being investigated as possible future migraine therapies.

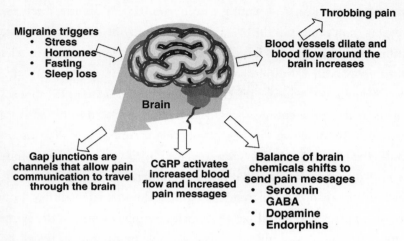

Mechanism of a migraine.

GETTING A DIAGNOSIS

There are no specific diagnostic tests such as X-rays or blood tests to tell if your headaches are migraines. A diagnosis of migraine is confirmed only after your doctor carefully examines your headache symptoms and history. She may decide you need to have tests to make sure your

There are no blood tests or X-rays that can specifically diagnose migraine. A careful history is the best approach.

headaches are not caused by some other medical condition. Most people with headaches won't need to have blood tests, X-rays, or special tests such as computed tomography scans (CT scans) or magnetic resonance imaging scans (MRI scans). These tests are usually reserved for patients whose headache histories or examinations suggest that their headaches are not typical migraines but may be due to other medical problems.

How Do I Know If My Headaches Are Migraine?

Migraine is diagnosed when your headache pattern is similar to those of other people with migraine. To see if your headaches might be migraine, answer the Migraine Questionnaire on page 22. If your answers to these questions don't suggest that your headaches might be caused by a medical problem other than migraine, take the ID Migraine Screener Quiz shown on page 23 to see if you might have migraine. If your headaches are a new medical problem, make sure you take the results of these questionnaires to your doctor to confirm a migraine diagnosis.

Track Your Headache Symptoms

Completing the daily headache diary on page 24 (or download it from www.diamedicapub.com) can be a great way to uncover your unique headache pattern. Reviewing this diary will be helpful for you and your doctor. A diary can help identify:

A daily headache diary is a good tool to help understand your unique headache pattern. Diaries help with diagnosis and identify early response to treatment.

► Whether your headache pattern is typical of migraine
► What triggers your headache
► Lifestyle changes you might implement to improve your headache
► Whether your headache pattern is changing
► Whether your headache is responding to prescribed treatments

You might also get headache diary applications for your electronic devices. For example, iHeadache is a headache tracking program that you can use on your iPhone, iPod Touch, and Blackberry. You can find out more at www.iHeadacheApp.com.

When Should I See My Doctor?

Be sure to seek medical attention if there is any doubt about the cause of your headaches or they are causing significant disability; for example, you're missing work or family activities. Remember—*migraines are*

MIGRAINE QUESTIONNAIRE

Answer these questions to see if you might have migraine

1. **Have you been having recurring headaches for several months?**
    Migraines are chronic headaches that often occur periodically for many
    years. If you have a new headache or new headache symptoms, be sure to
    see your doctor.

2. **Have you been having other health problems besides your headaches?**
    Headache is a common symptom of many medical conditions. If you're
    having other symptoms besides your headache, be sure to talk to your
    doctor.

3. **Did your headaches start after an illness or surgery, or within
    1 week of a head injury?**
    Headache may occur after illness or injury. Headaches commonly occur
    after head injuries with concussions. These post-trauma headaches can
    mimic migraines and should be evaluated by your doctor.

4. **How often do you take pain medications for your headaches?**
    Excessive use of over-the-counter and prescription painkillers can cause
    headaches to become more frequent, more severe, and more difficult to
    treat. Headaches that occur when you're regularly using pain medications
    3 or more days each week are called *analgesic overuse headaches* or *medica-
    tion overuse headaches*, and they need to be treated first by restricting pain
    medications. Migraine treatments typically won't work if you're also over-
    using pain medications.

5. **What do you prefer to do when you get a headache?**
    People with migraine often like to avoid stimulation—retreating to a dark,
    quiet room, for example. You might also notice that you're especially sen-
    sitive to odors and perfumes, and that your skin is sensitive to touch.

6. **Do your headaches limit your activities?**
    Migraine is a disabling headache, generally causing interference or disrup-
    tion of your daily routine. While you may need to stay at work when you
    have a migraine, you might find that you are less efficient, or you might
    prefer to cut back on evening activities after work because of a migraine.

ID MIGRAINE SCREENER QUIZ

Answer the following three questions about your headaches:

1. Over the last 3 months, have you limited your activities on at least 1 day because of your headaches?

2. Do lights bother you when you have a headache?

3. Do you get sick to your stomach or nauseated with your headache?

If you answered "yes" to at least two of these questions, you probably have migraine.

controllable. Be sure to talk to your doctor if you answered "yes" to any of the questions on page 25.

What Kind of Doctor Should I See?

Many different types of doctors treat patients with headaches:

- ▶ Primary care physicians
- ▶ Neurologists
- ▶ Headache specialists
- ▶ Gynecologists
- ▶ Dentists
- ▶ Ear, nose, and throat doctors

In most cases, primary care physicians such as family doctors or internists can effectively manage migraine. If you have failed to achieve good results with your primary care doctor, you may wish to see a neurologist or headache specialist. Links at the American Headache Society webpage (www.achenet.org) and National Headache Foundation website (www.headaches.org) can help you find a headache specialist in your area.

HEADACHE DIARY

Directions: Complete this diary three times every day—whether you have a headache on that day or not. Daily recording will help identify symptoms that predict when a headache will occur (prodrome) and the role of possible factors that might be triggering your migraines.

	SUN	MON	TUE	WED	THU	FRI	SAT
Pain severity 0=none 1=mild 2=moderate 3=severe							
Morning							
Afternoon							
Evening							
Triggers							
Menstrual day							
Skipped meals							
Poor sleep							
High stress							
Food (list)							
Weather							
Change							
Prodrome							
Fatigue							
Irritability							
Food cravings							
Neck pain							
Yawning							

WHEN TO SEE THE DOCTOR

Answer these questions to see if you should see your doctor about your headaches:

1. Are you unsure of your headache diagnosis, or what's causing your headaches?

2. Has there been a change in your headache pattern, frequency, or severity?

3. Have you developed a new type of headache?

4. Have you developed new health problems? Or are you worried that your headache or its treatment might affect another medical condition you have?

5. Do you think your headache treatment is not working?

6. Are you having trouble with your headache medication or unusual side effects?

7. Are you unsure what to do when you get a headache or how to take your medication?

8. Are you unsure about what you can do to help prevent headaches?

9. Do your headaches interfere with your daily routine, work, or family or social activities?

10. Do you avoid activities for fear you'll get a headache?

If you answered "yes" to any of these questions, be sure you talk to your doctor.

What Should I Do Before I See the Doctor?

Maintaining a headache diary and paying attention to your unique headache patterns can provide good information for you to take to your doctor. Be prepared to answer the following questions:

1. When did your headaches begin?
2. How long have your headaches been the way they are now?
3. How often do you get headaches?
4. How long does each headache episode last?
5. Do you have any warning symptoms that a headache is going to happen?

6. What have you done in the past to treat the headache? Did it work?
7. Do headaches run in your family? Do your mom, dad, sisters/brothers, or children have headaches?
8. Are other symptoms associated with the headache? Are you sensitive to noises, lights, or odors? Do you get sick to your stomach?
9. Are the headaches bad enough to make you miss work, go home from school, or miss out on family activities?
10. Have you been evaluated for headaches in the past? Were any tests ordered?
11. Does anything in particular bring on your headaches?
12. Have your headaches occurred around your menses or at mid-cycle? Did they change during pregnancy?
13. Do you have any other medical conditions or health symptoms?
14. What medications (over-the-counter, prescription, and natural remedies, supplements, or vitamins) do you use? What do you take when you get a headache?

The answers to these questions will help your doctor make the proper diagnosis.

What Should You Expect from Your Doctor's Office Visit?

There are many things that can come out of a visit to the doctor about your headaches. Don't expect to get all of your questions answered in one visit. You will probably need to work with your healthcare provider over several visits to refine your particular treatment strategy. You should expect to learn the answers to these questions:

1. What's my diagnosis, and what's causing my headaches?
2. Is my healthcare provider comfortable treating this headache condition?
3. Do I need further testing?

4. What medications will help my symptoms during a headache attack?
5. Do I need a medication for nausea?
6. Do I need to take preventive medication?
7. Are there other treatments that don't involve medications that can help my headaches?
8. What if I become pregnant?
9. Where can I learn more about headaches?
10. When should I come back?

You will find general answers to many of these questions throughout this book. Your healthcare provider can help clarify what you might expect in your individual situation.

Summary

Migraine is a very common, controllable, symptom complex that involves headache, nausea, and light sensitivity. It is often inherited, and it has a biological basis.

▶ One in every six women has migraines.
▶ Migraine is a biological condition caused by changes in nerves and blood vessels around the brain. Migraine is also a *threshold disorder*, meaning that some people are born with a brain that is more susceptible to migraine triggers. Some people are just more prone to headaches than others—even within the same family.
▶ Migraine is a complex process that may include up to four phases. Understanding the characteristics of each phase will allow you to identify symptoms that suggest you can treat your migraine early, before severe symptoms begin.

▶ A daily diary is a good tool to help record your individual headache symptoms, so that you can better understand your unique headache pattern.

▶ Reviewing this diary will help clarify your headache diagnosis, suggest possible interventions and the timing of treatment, and show early changes after you've started a treatment regimen.

The *good* news is that there are many things you can do to help relieve your migraines. Now that you understand more about migraines, you're ready to learn what you can do to help control them. As you learn more about both medication and non-medication treatments, remember the biological changes that happen during migraine, so that you understand how and why these treatments will be helpful.

2

Headaches from Puberty to Menopause

Hormones, Hormones, and More Hormones

Migraine often changes as women move through their reproductive lifecycle. Although many of us may think of being pregnant as our reproductive time, reproductive changes actually begin at puberty and continue through menopause. Hormone levels fluctuate during each of these stages, and these changes in hormones often result in significant variations in headache patterns as women move into puberty, start having monthly menstrual periods, use different contraceptives, have children, breastfeed, and eventually experience menstrual irregularities in the early stages of menopause, and finally experience the end of menses with later menopause.

Migraine typically affects people in their late teens and young adulthood, although it also occurs in childhood and later adulthood. Before puberty, migraine is far less common, typically affecting about 5 percent of children, with boys affected slightly more often than girls. Once puberty begins, hormones, especially estrogen, play a major role in the development of headaches. Changes in headache patterns occur predictably in many girls and women, with headache changes linked to changing levels of hormones. Because of the important relationship between hormones and headaches, this chapter reviews the hormonal changes that occur during a woman's reproductive life, and how they can relate to changes in headache patterns. Treatment options during different lifecycle changes will be covered in later chapters.

HORMONES PLAY A KEY ROLE IN HEADACHE DEVELOPMENT, ESPECIALLY IN WOMEN

What Exactly Is a Hormone?

Hormones are chemical substances that are made by cells in one part of the body, and then released to control and regulate different cells, often in other parts of the body. Hormones can be stored in organs called *glands* and released later, when needed. Hormones perform a wide range of important functions. They can affect growth, development, and reproduction, as well as regulate the body's metabolism, immune system, and mood. As noted in the table on page 31, a wide variety of hormones are produced in many parts of the body. The sex hormones play the most significant role in migraine.

What Are the Sex Hormones?

Sex hormones in women are produced by the ovaries and adrenal glands, and in men by the testes. There are several important sex hormones:

- ▶ Estrogens
- ▶ Progesterone
- ▶ Androgens, such as testosterone

You might be surprised to know that sex hormones are made from cholesterol, which also makes vitamin D. Did you ever wonder why good food sources for vitamin D (such as fatty fish, egg yolks, and butter) are also rich in cholesterol? When planning your diet, remember

IMPORTANT HORMONES IN THE BODY

Hormone	Where It's Produced	What It Does
Cholecystokinin	Small intestine	Releases digestive enzymes
Erythropoietin	Kidneys	Makes red blood cells
Growth hormone	Pituitary gland	Growth
Insulin	Pancreas	Controls metabolism of carbohydrates and fats
Leptin	Fat cells	Controls appetite and fat metabolism
Melatonin	Pineal gland in the brain	Regulates sleep
Renin	Kidneys	Adjusts blood pressure
Sex hormones	Mainly ovaries, testes, and adrenal glands	Affects reproductive development
Thyroid hormone	Thyroid gland	Affects body temperature, heart rate and blood pressure, metabolism, and weight

that it's important to include some cholesterol in a healthy meal plan. Too much cholesterol is bad, but so is not enough!

The female sex hormone *estrogen* has three components:

▶ *Estradiol*—the most potent naturally occurring estrogen; abundant in younger women, with levels declining during menopause
▶ *Estriol*—the primary estrogen produced by the placenta during pregnancy
▶ *Estrone*—the primary estrogen produced during menopause

Estrogen has important effects on female reproductive development, bone health, cardiovascular well-being, and brain function. It also has important effects on pain signal transmission, making it the most important sex hormone that affects headaches.

Progesterone prepares the uterus for pregnancy and helps to maintain a healthy pregnancy. The word *progestogen* refers to any hormone compound that affects the uterus, such as naturally occurring progesterone. Synthetic versions of progesterone are called *progestins*. For example, the compounds used to provide a progesterone effect in birth control pills are progestins.

Testosterone is thought of as the primary male hormone. In fact, there are several male hormones or *androgens*, which have important roles in the health of muscles, bone, and skin:

▶ *Dehydroepiandrosterone* (DHEA)—the main androgen for both men and women; DHEA is metabolized to form *testosterone* and *androstenedione*

▶ *Testosterone*—higher levels in men result in increased bone and muscle mass as compared with women

▶ *Androstenedione*—this compound breaks down into estrogens (estradiol and estrone) and testosterone

Although estrogens are thought of as female sex hormones and androgens are considered male hormones, both men and women make hormones in both groups, with different ratios depending on gender. For example, women make less than 10 percent of the amount of testosterone that men make. Testosterone is important in women for muscle and bone strength, and also for maintaining a healthy sex drive. Estrogen may play an important role in preventing heart disease in men. Younger men generally have higher levels of testosterone and lower levels of estrogen. With aging, estrogen levels often increase and testosterone levels decrease. This can lead to an increased risk of heart attacks, strokes, prostate enlargement, and prostate cancer in older men.

Even though sex hormones are important for good health, excessive hormone levels in either men or women can cause problems, so you shouldn't take extra hormones without supervision by your doctor.

DO KIDS HAVE SEX HORMONES?

Absolutely! Even though you usually hear about sex hormones for the first time at puberty, sex hormones are at work in children too. Puberty generally begins earlier in girls: 8–13 years old—and boys enter puberty between 10 and 15 years of age. With puberty, the brain signals the ovaries and testes to produce a variety of hormones that affect growth and development.

Sex hormones, however, are present in low concentrations in children before puberty, often at levels too low to be detected with the standard tests used during puberty and adulthood. Research has shown that estradiol levels are higher in girls than in boys, even before puberty. Some experts argue that a higher concentration of estradiol in girls results in earlier puberty. Sex hormones have been shown to affect bone growth and nerve development in children before puberty.

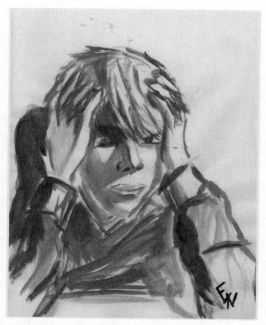

Migraines often affect both sides of the head in children.

The effect of hormones on headaches is also much more important after puberty. Once puberty begins, hormone levels increase and play a much more significant role in developing the physical changes that occur in boys and girls as they mature.

If Hormones Control Sexual Development, What Do They Have to Do with Pain?

Although we call estrogen, progesterone, and androgens *sex hormones*, they do more than just affect reproductive development. Sex hormones have strong influences on the brain and nervous system, and they have important roles in brain development and function. For example, estrogen affects both the anatomy and physiology of the part of the brain called the *hippocampus*. The hippocampus—from the Greek word for seahorse because of its shape—plays an important role in long-term memory, orientation, and navigation. This may explain why women are better at remembering anniversaries and have different ways of giving directions than men do. Because the hippocampus actually makes estrogens and androgens from cholesterol in the bloodstream, gender influences on the brain continue throughout our lifetimes. In Alzheimer's disease, the hippocampus is one of the first areas to be damaged. This results in the common early symptoms of Alzheimer's—memory loss and disorientation. Androgens and progesterone affect nerve functions less than estrogens.

You can think of the brain as though it's a giant communication network. Nerve cells in our brain and nervous system talk to each other by sending chemical messages from one nerve to the next. The places where communication between nerves occurs are called *synapses*, and these synapses sit on structures on the nerves called *dendritic spines*. The dendritic spines are like cell-phone holders of the nerves, with the synapses being the cell-phones ready to send and receive messages. Estrogen affects nerves by actually increasing the numbers of dendritic spines and synapses, making communication

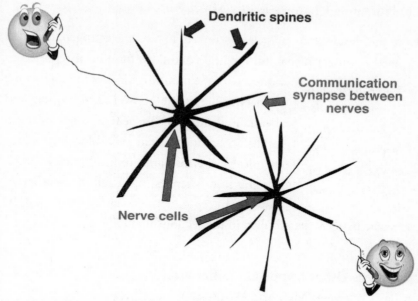

Headache messages are sent through complex networks of nerves. Communication points, called *synapses*, on nerve spines send signals from one nerve to the next until the brain is activated.

between neighboring nerves easier. (Didn't you already know women are great communicators?)

This enhanced communication network is thought to also make sending pain messages easier, which may explain why women are more sensitive to pain than men.

Sex hormones also influence the brain by affecting the levels of several important signaling chemicals, called *neurotransmitters*. The chemical messages they transmit amplify, relay, and change information across synapses from nerve to nerve. Estrogen, for example, directly affects the level and activity of both headache-producing (e.g., *dopamine* and *norepinephrine*) and headache-protecting (e.g., *serotonin, gamma amino-butyric acid* [GABA], and *endorphins*) neurotransmitters. In general, elevated estrogen increases headache protectors, reducing headache risk. Conversely, decreases in estrogen levels increase dopamine and norepinephrine, which in turn increase the chance of a headache occurring.

Do Hormone Changes *Really* Affect Pain Levels?

Pain threshold levels are clearly linked to cycling estrogen levels in women. A variety of painful medical conditions have been reported to

Estradiol enhances communication between nerves, accounting for the increased sensitivity to pain in women.

worsen with the monthly cycle, including chronic headaches, irritable bowel syndrome, and rheumatoid arthritis. In general, high estrogen results in an increase in pain-blocking neurochemicals, whereas pain-producing neurochemicals increase when estrogen falls to low levels. How each reproductive stage typically affects

headache patterns is described in the sections that follow.

Are There Other Important Differences in Pain Between Men and Women?

Men and women feel pain differently. Research studies consistently show that women are more sensitive to pain than men. They show that

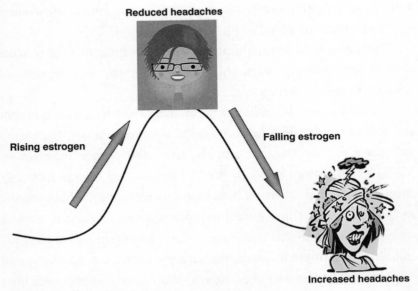

Effect of estrogen on headaches.

women feel pain at a lower stimulus than men, and pain becomes intolerable to women sooner than men.

▶ Women can *first* detect pain with a stimulus that's nearly 20 percent less than the stimulus needed for men to feel pain.

▶ Pain becomes *intolerable* with a stimulus that's 15 percent lower in women than men.

Similarly, studies also show that women find needle sticks and intravenous catheter placement to be more painful than men do.

Do Sex Hormones Affect Response to Pain Treatment?

Have you ever been frustrated when your male partner or friend tells you that a particular pain medication works great for him, looking at you a bit suspiciously when you say it doesn't help your pain at all? Unfortunately, many doctors are not aware that pain medications work differently for men and women.

To illustrate this, one research study showed that ibuprofen effectively reduced the threshold to experiencing experimental pain in men. In women, ibuprofen was no better than taking a sugar pill or *placebo*. In addition, certain narcotic painkillers (also called *opioids*) work better in men, while others work better in women. One class of narcotics, called *mu-opioids*, work better in men; morphine is an example of a mu-opioid.

Pain medications work differently for men and women.

One study comparing postoperative pain in men and women found that women required a 30 percent higher morphine dose to get pain relief than did men. Another class of narcotics, called *kappa-opioids*, work better in women; *butorphanol* is an example of a kappa-opioid that is often used during delivery to control labor pain or provide epidural anesthesia. Although it is not understood why gender differences occur, it is very clear that these differences are real. Estrogen is likely to be responsible for them.

HOW DO HORMONE LEVELS CHANGE OVER A WOMAN'S LIFETIME?

Estrogen levels change over a woman's lifetime in a predictable pattern. As estradiol levels rise and fall, migraines tend to become more frequent and severe. Puberty and the early stages of menopause (called the *perimenopause*) are two times in a woman's life when estradiol levels fluctuate quite a bit and, not surprisingly, an increase in headache activity also occurs. Smaller estradiol fluctuations occur with the monthly cycle, and greater fluctuations occur during pregnancy. Although headache patterns may temporarily change at these times, the overall headache *pattern* often continues to be relatively consistent until perimenopause, except during pregnancy.

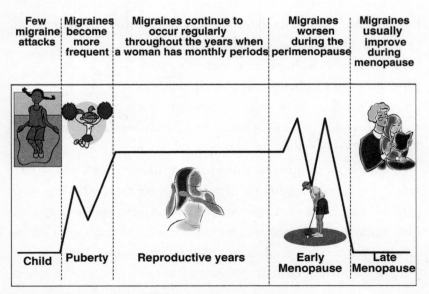

Typical changes in hormones and headaches over a lifetime.

What to Expect During Childhood and Adolescence

What Exactly Is Puberty and Why Is It Important?

During puberty, physical changes occur as the child moves into adulthood and becomes capable of reproduction. It is a monumental transition in the human lifecycle. The *gonads* (ovaries in girls and testes in boys) mature and release sex hormones, leading to important changes in the skin, brain, muscles, bones, and sex organs. *Adolescence* is the period between puberty and adulthood. In general, a *child* is anyone less than 12 years old, and an *adolescent* is anyone between 12 and 17 years old.

Prior to puberty, the physical differences between boys and girls are restricted to the genitalia. During puberty, a wide variety of changes result in significant physical differences between the sexes. Girls typically begin puberty 1–2 years before boys and also finish puberty sooner. They reach adult height and reproductive maturity on average about 4 years after puberty starts. Boys start puberty later, but generally continue to grow and mature for about 6 years after its onset.

In girls, changes in the breasts and genitalia generally begin around the ages of 10 or 11. The uterus and ovaries increase in size, and the ovaries begin to produce estrogen. *Menarche*, the onset of menstrual periods, starts about 1–2 years after breast changes begin. As estrogen levels increase, menstrual periods begin, and are accompanied by cycling estradiol levels. This is a critical factor in the development of headaches, because variations in estrogen levels are thought to be one of the most important drivers of migraine. At this stage, headaches become much more prominent in females than males.

Do Children Ever Get Migraines Before Puberty?

Headaches are relatively common in children. In one recent survey, headaches were reported by a significant number of children. Here are some interesting facts from this survey:

▶ Headaches occurred in the previous 6 months for four of every ten children.

▶ Migraines occurred in only 4 percent of children.

▶ Headaches started about 6 months earlier in boys than in girls.

With adolescence, headaches typically increase:

▶ Headaches occurred in the previous 6 months in six of every ten adolescents.

▶ Migraines occurred in 10 percent of adolescents.

Childhood and adolescent headaches are important to recognize and treat, because recurring headaches in children and adolescents often become chronic in adults. In addition, children with headaches are absent from school twice as often as children without them.

Headaches tend to disappear earlier in boys than in girls. In boys, migraines often stop before they leave the teenage years. Girls typically continue to have migraines throughout their reproductive years.

WHAT TO EXPECT WITH MENSES AND ORAL CONTRACEPTIVE USE

What Happens During Menses?

The menstrual cycle is necessary for reproduction. It typically is divided into the menstruation, follicular, and luteal phases. The length of each of these three phases can vary from woman to woman and from cycle to cycle. The average complete menstrual cycle is about 28 days.

During the *follicular phase*, estrogen gradually increases, and the lining of the uterus thickens. Follicles in the ovaries develop, each containing an ovum, or egg, waiting to be fertilized. After several days of development, one or two follicles continue to develop, while the others shrink and die.

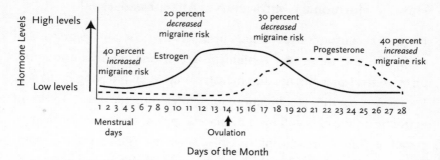

Estrogen (solid line) and progesterone (dashed line) levels change throughout the month. Both hormones are at their lowest levels during menstrual bleeding. Estrogen rises after menstrual bleeding and falls with ovulation. After ovulation, there is a marked increase in progesterone and a moderate increase in estrogen until your next menstrual period, when these hormones again drop to low levels. The risk of having a migraine increases around the time of menses and decreases between menses and ovulation.

About mid-cycle, a hormone called *luteinizing hormone* surges, signaling the beginning of the *luteal phase*. Increasing levels of luteinizing hormone cause the dominant follicle to release its egg. This is termed *ovulation*. After the egg is released, it lives for 24 hours or less if it is not fertilized. Once released, the rest of the follicle begins to produce the hormone progesterone. This hormone prepares the uterine lining for potential implantation to establish a pregnancy if the egg is fertilized. If implantation doesn't occur within 2 weeks, estrogen and progesterone levels drop. This causes the uterus to shed its lining, resulting in menstrual bleeding.

Headaches typically occur as estrogen levels fall—occasionally at ovulation or mid-cycle, but more consistently during the days immediately prior to the onset of menstrual bleeding, when estrogen levels fall precipitously. In one study, migraine activity and menses were monitored in 40 women not using hormonal contraception. Migraines were less likely to occur during those phases of the cycle when estradiol levels were increasing, and 40 percent more likely to occur when they dropped before menstrual flow. Ovulation was not linked to an increased risk for migraine activity.

How Do Hormonal Contraceptives Affect Headaches?

Hormonal contraceptives include products that combine estrogen and progestin, and those that contain progestin only. Oral contraceptive birth control pills disrupt the menstrual cycle by blocking ovulation. Estrogen-progestin combination pills often provide three weeks of active hormone pills, followed by placebo pills for a week. The drop in estradiol that occurs during this placebo week often triggers a menstrual headache. Headache cycling is less consistently linked with progestin-only contraceptives.

Interestingly, oral contraceptives may cause some women to start having migraines. Although most women with preexisting headaches will not notice any worsening after starting oral contraceptives, new-onset migraine is more likely to occur in women taking oral contraceptives, compared to those not using birth control pills. When migraines begin after starting birth control pills, they usually go away after discontinuing the medication, although improvement may take several months and does not occur for all women. *If you have new-onset aura after starting birth control pills, be sure to see your doctor.*

WHAT TO EXPECT WITH PREGNANCY AND DELIVERY

What Is the Relationship of Hormones to Pregnancy, and How Does This Affect Headaches?

Pregnancy is another monumental milestone in a woman's reproductive life and, not surprisingly, it has a huge impact on headaches. Once menses occur regularly, pregnancy is possible. When successful fertilization occurs, the fertilized egg is implanted in the uterus and a variety of hormones are produced, including *human chorionic gonadotropin*, or hCG, the substance that is measured by pregnancy tests. This surge in hormones is thought to be responsible for early pregnancy symptoms such as morning sickness. hCG stimulates the lining of the uterus to begin producing progesterone, which helps to provide nourishment for the developing embryo. The placenta is formed and connects the developing fetus to the uterus. Although the ovaries continue to produce estrogen early on, as pregnancy develops the placenta begins to produce estrogen as well. As the pregnancy progresses, estrogen, progesterone, and hCG levels increase significantly.

Sixty to seventy percent of women with migraine will have significant improvement in their headache patterns during the second and third trimesters.

Estrogen levels rise dramatically during pregnancy and drop precipitously after delivery. The figure below shows the expected changes in estrogen levels during each trimester and during the *postpartum* period after delivery. Compared to first-trimester levels, estrogen increases sixfold by the third trimester and then drops to almost undetectable levels after delivery.

Many women find that headaches improve as estrogen levels surge during pregnancy. Improvement usually begins at the end of the first trimester. This tends to continue throughout the remainder of pregnancy, while estrogen levels stay high. When the baby is born, estrogen levels drop and headache protection is lost, causing headaches to begin again.

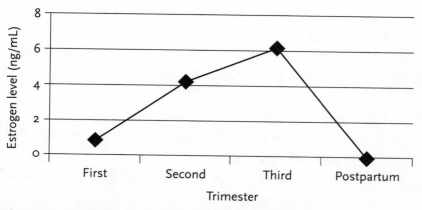

Changes in estrogen levels during pregnancy and after delivery.

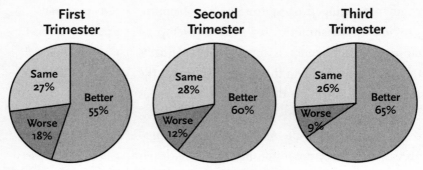

Expected changes in migraine activity with each trimester.

What If My Headaches Don't Go Away During Pregnancy?

Although most women experience headache improvement with pregnancy, some do not. These women may require more intensive treatment during pregnancy. In general, headaches improve by the end of the first trimester. If you're still having headaches at the time of your

Talk to your doctor if you're still having headaches when you go to your first visit with your obstetrician.

first obstetrical visit, they will likely continue during your pregnancy, and you should talk to your doctor about treatment options.

Some women actually develop their first migraine during pregnancy. *Although most headaches during pregnancy are not caused by serious health problems, you should talk to your doctor whenever you develop new headaches, notice a change in your headache pattern or symptoms, or note new health problems.* Some medical conditions that may cause headaches during pregnancy include:

- ▶ Infection
- ▶ *Preeclampsia/eclampsia* (high blood pressure, edema, and other complications of pregnancy)
- ▶ Brain vascular diseases (such as strokes, aneurysms, dissections, and vascular malformations)
- ▶ Brain tumors (especially pituitary *adenomas* and *meningiomas*)

▶ Increased intracranial pressure not related to tumors (called *pseudotumor* or *benign intracranial hypertension*)

Migraine sufferers are at increased risk for developing increased blood pressure with preeclampsia/eclampsia and strokes, although the overall occurrence of these complications is quite small. You can help reduce your risk of high blood pressure and strokes by following these healthy lifestyle habits:

▶ Avoid nicotine.
▶ Exercise regularly.
▶ Maintain normal levels of cholesterol in your diet.
▶ Avoid excess weight gain.

Will Having Headaches Hurt the Baby?

Women with migraines are not at increased risk for having a baby with birth defects or giving birth prematurely. Even women having severe migraines during their pregnancy generally have their babies born at full term and of similar weight as headache-free moms.

What Happens After I Deliver?

Even if headaches improve during pregnancy, they typically return during the first 1–4 weeks after delivery. As already noted, estrogen and progesterone levels remain high during the third trimester. Delivery of the placenta after the baby is born causes a sudden drop in progesterone and estrogen. Estrogen levels will remain low for the next several months. The drop in progesterone helps to stimulate the production of breast milk.

Nursing delays the return of migraines after delivery.

In most cases, headaches return to the pre-pregnancy pattern after delivery. If you choose to breastfeed, you're less likely to have your headache return during the first month after your baby is born.

NURSING DELAYS RETURN OF MIGRAINES AFTER DELIVERY		
	Number of moms for whom migraines have already returned	
Time after delivery	Breastfeeding	Bottlefeeding
1 week	2 in every 10 moms	8 in every 10 moms
1 month	4 in every 10 moms	Every mom

As a side note, it is recommended that women who breastfeed not take estrogen-containing birth control pills because the estrogen can decrease milk production.

WHAT TO EXPECT WITH MENOPAUSE

I'm done with my periods, and I still have headaches! My doctor said my headaches would go away once I hit menopause! What is going on here?

Menopause refers to the time in a woman's lifecycle when she has permanently stopped having her monthly menstrual periods. Menopause does not occur on a specific day; it's actually a long process. It is best thought of as a time of transition, beginning with the perimenopause and ending with the postmenopause.

The perimenopause is a time of marked hormonal change, usually beginning 6 or more months before menopause. Hormone levels fluctuate during perimenopause, resulting in menstrual irregularities, hot flashes, sweating, and other unpleasant symptoms. Menopause is officially diagnosed after a woman has gone 1 year without a menstrual period. Postmenopause refers to any time after menopause. Interestingly, women who experience an aura with their migraines are less likely to experience improvement with menopause than those whose migraines do not involve an aura.

Menopause occurs most commonly in Westernized countries at an average age of 51, with a typical range of 45 to 55 years of age. In some countries, such as in India and the Philippines, the average age of menopause is much lower, about 44 years old. The reason for this is unclear. Women who have had a hysterectomy and are thus unable to have menstrual periods can be diagnosed as reaching menopause with a blood test that measures the level of follicle-stimulating hormone or FSH, which increases during the menopause.

Headaches often worsen during the early part of menopause because of fluctuating estrogen levels.

Ovarian function decreases as women approach their late 40s, resulting in the diminished production of estrogen, progesterone, and testosterone. Initially, production becomes more irregular, with wide and unpredictable fluctuations in sex hormone levels. These wide hormonal fluctuations can result in typical perimenopausal symptoms, such as hot flashes, mood swings, and vaginal dryness. Migraines typically worsen as hormonal levels fluctuate during the perimenopausal period, and improvement is usually delayed until women reach the postmenopausal period. After the fluctuating estrogen levels have stabilized and estrogen production drops to consistently low levels, headaches usually lessen in the majority of women and often go away for good. (See—there is at least one benefit from menopause!)

If I Have a Hysterectomy, Will My Headaches Go Away?

Going through natural menopause results in migraine improvement for two of every three women. Women having a *hysterectomy* and *oophorectomy* (removal of the uterus and ovaries) will also go through menopause; however, their headaches are more likely to worsen. The unpredictable changes in headache pattern with fluctuating estrogen levels suggest that these patterns are complicated and affected by more than simply estrogen levels.

**After Spontaneous
Menopause**

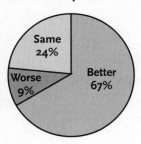

**After Surgical
Menopause (Hysterectomy)**

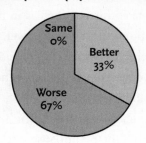

Changes in migraine with menopause.

Will Estrogen Medications Affect My Headaches?

Treatment of early menopausal symptoms with hormone replacement therapy may result in alterations in headache. However, studies have failed to show a consistent pattern of change with hormonal supplements, with women as likely to experience improvement or worsening of their headaches. One consistent finding, however, is that headaches are more likely to worsen in women treated with oral hormonal replacement, compared with transdermal hormone replacement using skin patches. Experts believe women experience a steadier dose of hormones with a transdermal patch, compared with oral pills, resulting in the better response.

SUMMARY

- ▶ Hormones play a key role in the development, improvement, and worsening of headaches during the reproductive life of women.
- ▶ Estrogens affect the anatomy and function of the brain and nerves, making women more sensitive to pain than men.
- ▶ Before puberty, boys have more headaches than girls; after puberty, girls get more headaches.

▶ Headaches in boys often stop during the teenage years or in early adulthood. Headaches in girls often continue until menopause.

▶ Headaches generally worsen with cycling estrogen, with increased headache activity during menstrual bleeding and during the placebo week of birth control pills.

▶ Headaches typically improve at the end of the first trimester of pregnancy. Women who continue to have problematic headaches at the end of the first trimester usually continue to have headaches throughout the rest of their pregnancy.

▶ Although headaches often worsen during the months before menstrual periods completely stop (perimenopause), they generally improve in the postmenopausal period.

3

Migraine Management

What Really Works?

Now that we have an overview of what happens during a migraine and some of the factors that influence whether a migraine will occur or not, let's move on to the crucial question: *How do you manage migraines? What really works?* The good news is that many treatments effectively reduce headache frequency and severity, but the bad news is that there's no quick fix or migraine cure.

Monitoring your headaches will give you important information. Understanding your personal headache pattern is essential when choosing which treatments are most appropriate for you. For example, you'll need to use more aggressive treatment if your headaches start out severe and disabling or are maximum upon awakening, as compared with women whose headaches begin as milder pain progressing to a more disabling headache over time. Logging your headaches can also provide clues about when you are most susceptible—for example, around your period. This information can help you develop a headache strategy that will work best for your pattern.

LEARNING ABOUT YOUR HEADACHE THRESHOLD

What Is a Headache Threshold, and Why Is It Important?

Everyone has a different threshold for getting a headache. If you have a low headache threshold, you're very likely to get headaches; if you have a high threshold, you're less likely to get them. Understanding the concept of an individual headache threshold helps explain why some people are bothered by more troublesome headaches than others

Let's use nitroglycerin as an example. Nitroglycerin is a very potent blood vessel dilating medication and a potent headache trigger. Taking it will produce headaches in almost everyone—including people who rarely get them—but people who are headache-prone will develop one at a much lower dose. Less potent triggers, such as eating certain foods, skipping a meal, sleeping late, having your menstrual period, or having a stressful day, can also provoke a headache in susceptible people. Therefore, people with a low headache threshold may get a headache after a stressful day or drinking one glass of red wine, but those with a high headache threshold won't.

People with a high headache threshold may find that they need to have a combination of several triggers occurring together before they get a headache. For this reason, you may find that you sometimes get a headache when you drink red wine, but only if you also are having your menstrual period *and* had a stressful day at work. Changes in your body may change your headache threshold on a day-to-day basis, so you may find that some days you have a lower threshold and are more prone to developing a headache after experiencing headache triggers than on other days when your threshold is higher.

How Do I Figure Out My Threshold?

The best way to learn more about your headache threshold is to keep a headache diary. This will help you begin to identify the consistent circumstances that are present when you have a headache. You'll probably need to

Person with a LOW headache threshold

Headache occurs when exposed to a single trigger

Person with a HIGH headache threshold

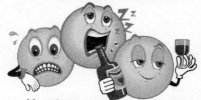

Headache only occurs after exposure to several triggers

What's needed to trigger a headache—understanding headache threshold.

keep a diary for several weeks or months in order to identify consistent patterns with your headaches. You can use the diary on page 24 to begin logging your headache activity. Reviewing your diary can help you better understand your headache threshold. You can then understand what specific triggers, under what circumstances, can bring on a headache.

How Can I Raise My Headache Threshold?

Non-drug and medication prevention therapies both work by raising the headache threshold—making it harder for you to get a headache. Individuals with low thresholds are excellent candidates for preventive therapy. Those with a higher threshold may use prevention therapy when they expect to be exposed to those triggers to which they are sensitive, such as during their menstrual periods. People with low thresholds may also need to increase their preventive strategies at times when they can predict they will be more likely to be exposed to headache triggers, such as when traveling, at times of high stress, and around the menstrual period.

Because all effective preventive medications raise the headache threshold, several treatment options can be used at once, providing an additive effect. When a particularly bad headache occurs, or a consistently bad time in the month is noted, a higher dose of the preventive medication or combination of preventive therapies (such as medications and non-medication options) may be needed to effectively raise the threshold.

NON-DRUG TREATMENT OPTIONS

I don't want to rely on drugs. What are my options?

Non-drug treatments generally help prevent headaches by raising the headache threshold. Some non-drug treatments, such as relaxation, biofeedback, and physical therapy exercises, may also be used to treat an individual headache episode. Non-drug treatments reduce brain pain chemicals, relax muscles, and decrease stress hormones, such as adrenaline. The obvious advantage of non-drug treatment is that you don't have to worry about medication side effects.

Who Might Benefit Most from Non-Drug Treatments?

Everyone who suffers from headaches can benefit from non-drug treatment options. Even people who use medications will find they get better headache relief when they combine drugs with non-drug therapies. Non-drug treatments may be particularly helpful for people who need to restrict prescription medications to minimize troublesome side effects, such as:

▶ Women who are pregnant or breastfeeding
▶ Children and adolescents
▶ People who prefer not to take medications
▶ People who are unable to take or tolerate certain medications
▶ People who are treating other health problems with drugs that might interact with migraine medications

Individuals who are not in any of these groups, as well as those who use some migraine medications, may also improve their headache relief by adding non-drug treatments to their regimen. Headache treatment does not need to be only medications or only non-drugs. In many cases, combining effective treatments from both categories will enhance your relief. Research studies have shown that people taking medications do best when they add effective non-drug treatments to their medication treatments.

Furthermore, patients using medication prevention and non-drug treatments can often discontinue medicines after their headaches have been controlled for about 6 months. Researchers believe this long-lasting benefit after drugs have been discontinued can be attributed to a combination of balancing brain chemicals and maintaining this balance through continued use of non-drug therapies.

Which Non-Drug Treatments Really Work?

There are many non-drug treatment options for headache. The most effective ones are:

- ▶ Relaxation with or without biofeedback
- ▶ Stress management
- ▶ Cognitive restructuring
- ▶ Distraction techniques
- ▶ Exercises
- ▶ Acupressure
- ▶ Healthy lifestyle habits

Relaxation and Biofeedback

Relaxation techniques are among the most effective headache prevention therapies. They work by activating pain-relieving centers in the brain. Relaxation training produces changes in serotonin levels similar to those that occur when taking typical prescription headache medications. So, it's not just a matter of "chilling out" to relieve your headaches; you're actually learning how to control the release of pain-provoking and pain-relieving brain chemicals using specific, easy-to-learn techniques.

Relaxation can be taught using several techniques:

▶ Visual imagery
▶ Deep-breathing techniques
▶ Progressive muscle relaxation
▶ Biofeedback

Visual imagery is a technique in which an individual imagines a calm, pleasurable scene or experience and focuses just on that image. If the mind wanders, the individual guides it back to focusing on the pleasurable image. Deep-breathing exercises and progressive muscle relaxation are two other ways to achieve relaxation.

Biofeedback is a type of relaxation that uses biological measures—such as your finger temperature, respiratory rate, or muscle tone—to tell you if you've successfully achieved a relaxed state—hence the name *bio* (for biological) and *feedback* (meaning information that tells you how you're doing). Biofeedback can include complex computerized

---

VISUAL IMAGERY

▶ Go to a quiet, dimly lit room where you won't be disturbed.

▶ Close your eyes.

▶ Begin to recall a place where you have been or would like to be.

▶ As you focus on the scene, slowly add details about the experience.

▶ For example, you may think, "I am on a warm beach in Florida, lying on the warm sand, basking in the warm sun and listening to the relaxing waves of the ocean a short distance away. I can hear sea gulls flying about overhead. The smell of the salty water is pleasing."

▶ If your mind wanders, remind yourself, "I'm going back to the beach, where I'm lying on the warm sand and basking in the warm sun."

monitors of muscle contraction with graphic displays that provide feedback about muscle tension, or simple hand-held thermometers designed to demonstrate a few degrees increase in hand temperature when relaxation has been achieved (to about 96 degrees Fahrenheit, or 35–36 degrees Celsius). No single relaxation technique is more effective in reducing headaches than another, although some people prefer one specific technique or another. In general, biofeedback can be taught by a trained therapist in five or six treatment sessions, with additional practice needed at home between sessions. Once you've mastered these skills, you will

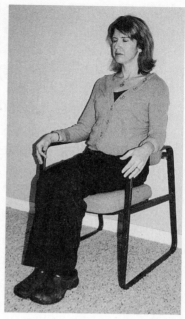

Proper posture for practicing relaxation techniques.

no longer have to practice daily, but only when you feel stressed or start to get a headache.

Relaxation techniques are perhaps the best-studied of non-drug treatments for migraine. Decades of research studies have proven that relaxation is very effective for raising the headache threshold and preventing headaches. In one study, headache activity was compared in 192 patients treated with relaxation training or *propranolol* (Inderal®), a standard migraine prevention drug. After 6 months, headache frequency, duration, and severity decreased by about half each for both treatment groups. Then patients were told to stop practicing relaxation techniques or taking propranolol. Six months later, headaches had worsened by at least half in 39 percent of those who had been treated with propranolol, but only 9 percent in the people trained to use relaxation. Researchers thought that migraine sufferers who knew how to use relaxation would likely continue to use the skills as needed after dis-

RELAXATION TECHNIQUES

▶ Relaxation techniques should be done while sitting in a comfortable chair, with arms and legs uncrossed, feet flat on the floor, and eyes closed. Alternatively, you can lie flat on the floor on your back with your hands comfortably lying across your chest.

▶ Each practice session should last for about 15–20 uninterrupted minutes.

▶ Once you have regularly practiced and mastered these techniques, you will be able to use them whenever you feel yourself starting to get tense, in anticipation of stress, or at the start of a headache.

▶ Effective techniques are *progressive muscle relaxation, cue-controlled relaxation*, and *thermal biofeedback*.

Progressive muscle relaxation consists of alternatively contracting and relaxing muscles throughout your body

▶ Close your eyes and practice tensing and then relaxing individual muscles in different parts of your body, starting at your feet and moving toward your neck and face.

▶ Hold the tension for 10–15 seconds and then release it.

▶ Tense and release the muscles in your legs, and then abdomen, arms, shoulders, neck, jaw, eyes, and finally forehead.

▶ Focus on how the muscles feel when they are no longer tensed.

▶ When you are familiar with this exercise, you will begin to recognize when your muscles are unusually tense, even if you don't feel "stressed." For example, you might notice jaw and neck tightness when sitting in traffic or waiting in a line at the store. When you become aware of this tightness, work to relax it as you do during your quiet training sessions.

Cue-controlled relaxation is a combination of deep breathing and repetition of the word "relax"

▶ While you can perform this activity seated, many find that it is easier to do while lying flat on your back on the floor.

▶ Begin this exercise with a slow, deep, abdominal breath.

▶ Place your hand over your abdomen to make sure that it is moving in and out with each breath. After breathing in, hold your breath for 5–10 seconds, and then breathe out, slowly repeating the word "relax." Repeat.

▶ After you are comfortable with this method, you should be able to close your eyes and take a deep breath as above before dealing with stressful situations, such as a doctor's visit, a meeting with the boss, or a discussion with your spouse. This will relax your system and reduce the effect of stressful situations on your pain-provoking mechanisms and headaches.

Thermal biofeedback uses finger temperature to identify your state of relaxation.

▶ Place a handheld thermometer on your finger and measure the temperature.

▶ Focus on raising your finger temperature by 2–3 degrees Fahrenheit (preferably to about 96 degrees) while practicing relaxation techniques.

▶ Some people find that it's difficult to "feel" relaxed. Using biofeedback can help show you when you are getting relaxed. Turning on and turning off specific pathways in your brain and nervous system will result in a feeling of calm, higher skin temperatures, and—most importantly—blocking of pain messages.

▶ An inexpensive finger thermometer and biofeedback audiotape can be obtained from Primary Care Network (1-800-769-7565).

▶ This is the same concept behind the "mood rings" of the 1960s. When the person was stressed, blood flow in the finger decreased resulting in a certain color such as red. With a more relaxed mood, the blood flow in the finger increases, resulting in a different color such as blue.

continuing daily practice, resulting in continued headache control for most of them.

Stress Management

Stress is the most commonly reported headache trigger. About three of every four headache sufferers identify stress as one of their headache triggers. Exposure to stress results in painful muscle contraction, as well as changes in pain chemicals in the nervous system—such as serotonin, endorphins, norepinephrine, and dopamine—that result in a lowered headache threshold.

Stress management is not a recommendation to eliminate exposure to stressful situations. Everyone's life is full of stress—including minor stresses such as confronting traffic or waiting in line at the store, and major stresses such as moving, having children, or facing the death of a loved one. Although exposure to these stresses cannot be eliminated, you can learn to change your body's response to stress.

Stress management teaches your body to react to stresses in different ways that do not result in the release of pain-provoking chemicals and tightening muscles. When you're stuck in aggravating city traffic on your way to an appointment, instead of experiencing a flare in temper, clenching your teeth, and tightening the muscles in your neck, you can repeat soothing thoughts, such as "I will make my appointment. I am a responsible person." You could listen to music while practicing relax-

---

FIND OUT IF STRESS IS MAKING YOUR HEADACHES WORSE

1. Do at least half of your headaches occur during or after a stressful day?

2. When you get a headache, do you feel powerless to help yourself get better?

3. Are you so busy with your job, family, and other commitments that you don't have time for activities you enjoy, such as hobbies, exercising, or meditation?

4. Do you feel like you'll never be able to catch up on your work or chores?

5. Have you had any major life changes (moving, marriage, job change, or loss of a close friend or family member) during the last year?

6. Do you wait until bedtime to finally start relaxing?

If you answered "yes" to any of these questions, stress may be making your migraines worse, and you should add stress management techniques to your treatment.

ation techniques such as slow, deep breathing. These same strategies can be used before attending a meeting with your boss or a child's teacher, before beginning a discussion about family issues with a spouse or child, or when waiting in a long line at the grocery store.

A 2-month treatment program compared headache reduction after treatment with stress management to using standard doses of the migraine prevention drug amitriptyline (Elavil®). Headache reduction was greater with stress management training (58 percent) compared

---

STRESS MANAGEMENT

▶ *Learn good time management.* Schedule a reasonable amount of activities, chores, or goals for each day. Overloading your schedule will inevitably result in a stress response:

- Write down which activities must be completed each day and delegate chores among members of your household.

- Accept that life won't be perfect. It's more important to have a relaxed home than a spotless one.

- Don't be afraid to say no. You can't volunteer for every worthwhile cause, and your kids don't need to participate in every possible after-school activity. Prioritize what's important for you and your family. Research shows that the healthiest volunteering is limited to no more than 2 hours per week.

- Schedule "down time" every day for reading, reflection, or a fun family activity.

▶ *Identify your stress buttons.* Learn what events typically make you feel stressed. You might be stressed after meeting with your boss, helping with a school project, or talking with your mother-in-law:

- Anticipate when your stress buttons will be pushed, and practice relaxation techniques beforehand.

- Stretch muscles when they first become tense.

- Provide positive encouraging messages to yourself before the beginning of a stressful activity to reduce your stress response.

STRESS MANAGEMENT (CONTINUED)

▶ *Practice daily "stress-busting."*

- Recognize and accept stressful events you can't control, such as the weather or other people's attitudes and behavior.

- Plan for stress by recognizing when stressful events are most likely to occur.

- Practice relaxation techniques and cognitive restructuring before encountering stress.

- Ask for help from others—you don't have to do everything yourself!

- Do aerobic exercise every day.

- Consider learning and practicing yoga, Tai Chi, and/or mindfulness meditation.

- Eat regularly—don't skip meals.

- Get plenty of sleep.

- Sing and find humor in your day.

---

with amitriptyline (33 percent). Patients who combine stress management with their usual drug therapies can expect the best reduction in their headaches. A variety of stress-management resources are listed in the Resource Guide at the end of this book. Many people find that working with someone who specializes in stress management is more effective than learning stress-relieving techniques on their own. Stress is everywhere, but our reactions to stress can be modified from negative reactions that increase headaches to positive coping techniques.

Cognitive Restructuring

Cognitive restructuring is a way of changing your thoughts from negative to positive. Negative thoughts about your headache include catastrophic thinking that the pain will never improve, that nothing you do will ever help, and that achieving pain relief is hopeless. More positive

▶ *Make realistic goals about your headaches.* Don't expect your treatment to cure your headaches. Realistic goals include achieving decreases in:

- Headache severity
- Headache frequency
- Headache duration
- Interference with life activities because of headaches
- Reliance on medications

▶ *Give yourself positive messages about your headaches:*

- "I can use skills I have learned to improve my headache."
- "My headache is going to get better."
- "I will continue to use relaxation and stress management techniques to help reduce my headache threshold."
- "I know what to do to treat my headaches."

▶ *Treat your headaches with positive behaviors:*

- During a headache, use active treatments like relaxation techniques, aerobic exercise, stretching, and ice packs.
- Avoid passive behaviors like retreating to a dark quiet room and lying in bed. While seeking quiet isolation may be necessary for severe headache episodes, active behaviors can provide important distractions during milder attacks to prevent escalation to more severe and incapacitating headaches.

self-messages might include thoughts about how pain management skills can help reduce your headache, that the headache will improve, and that you can change your behavior to reduce future headaches—for example, by practicing stress management before an anticipated stressful day. Working with a behavioral psychologist can help you master this skill.

Distraction Techniques

Your brain can only focus on so many things at once. For example, it's hard to balance your checkbook when your toddler's running around, the teenager's negotiating for more time with the family car, and the television's blaring in the other room. When a headache is still mild, you can often reduce your pain by distracting your brain with other, non-pain messages. While distracting behaviors will not necessarily control every headache, they can help maintain function, reduce focusing on headache symptoms, and decrease the likelihood of pain escalation. Surely you've heard of stage performers who are able to distract their brain from painful stimuli—for example, by walking on hot coals or lying on a bed of sharp nails! You don't have to be a stage performer to distract yourself from painful sensations. Most of us do this subconsciously as we work through our headaches.

DISTRACTION TECHNIQUES

You have probably been told to go to a dark, quiet room as soon as your headache starts. Unfortunately, if you do this, there will be nothing to distract your brain from headache pain messages, and your headache will probably get worse. You're more likely to keep your headache from becoming severe if you can distract your brain from focusing on pain signals. Unless your headache symptoms are severe, try to get involved in pleasant, distracting activities when your headache first begins, such as:

▶ Go outside for a brisk walk or gentle swim.

▶ Listen to soothing music.

▶ Perform stretching exercises.

▶ Use relaxation techniques.

▶ Apply ice to your neck.

These distracting behaviors can often help keep a headache mild or help get rid of it faster than by lying in bed.

Exercises

Four out of every five people with headaches have problems with neck posture and tender muscles in the head, neck, and shoulder that are probably aggravating their headaches. They often experience what is diagnosed as *myofascial pain syndrome*. This means the muscles become tight and tender, and may even cause shooting pains when pressed. Therapies to reduce headaches by improving abnormal muscle tension include:

▶ Myofascial or physical therapy
▶ Aerobic exercise
▶ Stretching exercises such Tai Chi, yoga, and Pilates

In one study, doing aerobic exercise three times per week for 6 weeks resulted in a nearly 45 percent reduction in headache severity.

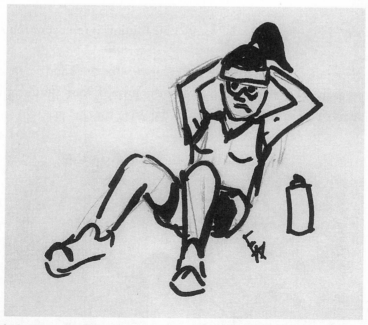

Muscle spasm can trigger migraines. Conditioning muscles to reduce muscle spasm can help reduce migraine activity.

▶ *Stretching exercises should be relaxing.* They should be done twice daily, with each session lasting about 15 minutes. Stretches should result in a normal sensation of stretching, but not pain. Hold the stretch for 5 seconds, relax for 5–10 seconds, and then repeat each stretch about 3–5 times.

▶ *If you have a headache, try doing these exercises in the shower or in a warm bath,* or after putting a heating pad on your neck for 15 minutes. Put ice packs on your neck after finishing stretching.

Stretching exercises targeting the neck and shoulder girdle may be used daily to help reduce headache frequency. Stretching during a mild headache can also help reduce pain and prevent the headache from becoming more severe. People with substantial neck pain or muscle tightness may benefit from an evaluation and treatment by a physical therapist.

Daily stretches. Practice a daily stretching routine to relax your muscles.

▶ *Neck range of motion.* Bend your chin to your chest and rotate chin to each shoulder. Then tip your ear toward your shoulder, and finally pull in your chin to make a double chin.

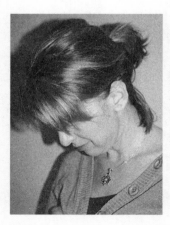 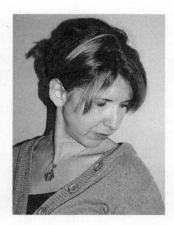

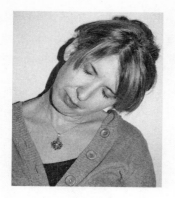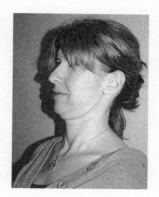

▶ *Shoulder shrugs.* Sit or stand up straight and raise your shoulders straight up. Lower and relax. Then raise shoulders up and forward. Lower and relax. Then raise shoulders up and back.

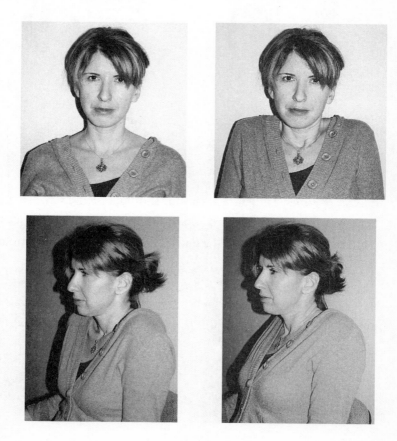

▶ *Suboccipital range of motion.* Place a rolled or folded towel behind your neck and gently pull down. Tilt your chin to your chest. Then look up at the ceiling. Then tilt your ear toward each shoulder.

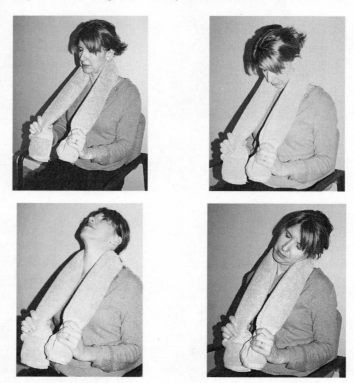

▶ *Neck stretches.* Tilt your ear to your shoulder on the same side, and then tilt your chin forward and toward the opposite breast. Gently press with your hand at the end of the stretch to feel the stretch.

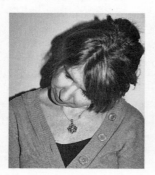
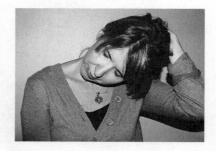

▶ *Neck isometrics.* Place your palm on your forehead and press your head against it, keeping you palm stationary. Don't let your head or hand move. Repeat with your hand on each side of your head.

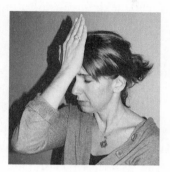

▶ *Head lift.* Place your folded hands behind your neck at the base of your head. Pull your elbows forward and up to achieve the sensation of lifting your head up slightly from your neck.

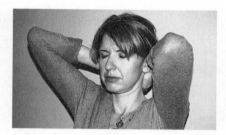

▶ *Turtle.* While looking forward, push the chin forward, away from your neck. When your head is forward, turn about 1 inch to each side and up.

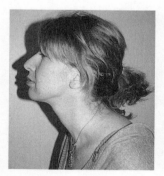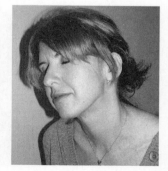

Stretching in the morning and before bed can help relieve stress before starting the day and aid in relaxation before sleep. Alternatively, you might do stretching exercises while watching your favorite daily television programs or while taking your morning shower.

Exercises to do during a headache episode. Apply heat or ice (whichever you find more soothing) for 20 minutes to your neck and shoulders. Then do the stretching exercises that you normally find the most soothing.

▶ *Oscillatory movements.* Make small, rhythmic, side-to-side head movements. While facing forward, turn your head slightly to one side and then back to forward. Repeat, going slowly back and forth at a rate of about once per second, for about 30 seconds. Rest for 30 seconds; then repeat until no further relief is noted. Then switch to turning the head toward the other side and proceed as above.

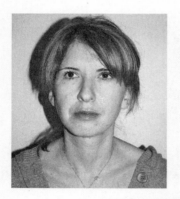 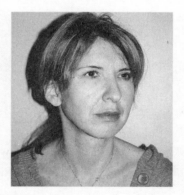

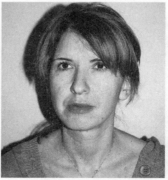

▶ *Positional distraction.* Place books on the floor in a 1- to 2-inch stack. Lie down on the floor, with the back of your head resting on the books. The edge of the books should be near the middle of your head, so your neck is free. Relax so that your head moves up from your neck. Avoid exercises (such as this one) that require you to lie on your back after the first trimester of pregnancy, because this position can put excess pressure on your blood vessels and reduce the blood flow going to your baby.

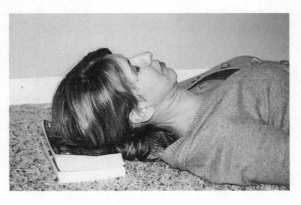

Trigger-Point Compression.   During a headache, you may notice certain spots on your muscles that aggravate your head pain when you press them. These are called *trigger points.* When you identify your trigger points, apply pressure to them with your fingers and hold for 15–60 seconds. Release the pressure and proceed with your usual stretching exercises. If these spots are hard to reach, try lying on a tennis ball placed under the trigger point, or use a Thera Cane® (www.theracane.com/)— a curved cane with knobs placed to help you get to hard-to-reach trigger points.

Postural Correction.   The human body was developed to be in perfect balance. Muscles on the left balance muscles on the right. Muscles in the front balance muscles in the back. When this balance is upset or one set of muscles is dominant, the resulting muscle imbalance often results in pain. Try to maintain your head in a neutral position with your ear lobes centered over the middle of each collarbone. Consciously try to get back to this position when you're standing in the grocery line, at the computer, or sitting in a class.

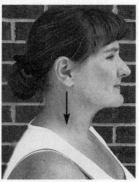

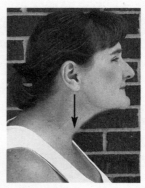

Balanced head posture with ear lobe over the middle of the collar bone.

Abnormal and unbalanced forward head posture with ear lobe in front of the collar bone.

Acupressure

Acupressure and acupuncture both work by activating specific points to help reduce pain symptoms. Acupuncture may be useful during an acute severe headache episode, especially if it is associated with tight neck and upper back muscles. While acupuncture is often helpful for other types of chronic pain, it is generally less helpful for people with chronic headache.

Healthy Lifestyle Habits

Headache sufferers consistently find that changes in their schedules or routines frequently trigger their headaches. Maintaining a healthy lifestyle can be an effective way to help raise the headache threshold. The most important lifestyle tips include:

- ▶ Sticking to a regular sleep schedule
- ▶ Not skipping meals
- ▶ Avoiding nicotine

ACUPRESSURE

Acupressure may be soothing when performed during a headache episode. Relief will be greatest if acupressure is followed by other pain-relieving therapies, such as relaxation techniques or stretching exercises.

▶ Find the depression in the middle of the back of your neck between the neck muscles, and move up within this depression to where the neck meets the skull. Firmly rub the area where the neck muscles attach to the skull for 2–3 minutes with deep circular movements.

▶ Find the depression at each temple, immediately behind your eyebrows. Rub firmly and deeply for 1 minute.

▶ Find the depression between your eyebrows. Rub firmly and deeply for 1 minute.

▶ Find the muscle that lies in the web between your thumb and index finger by compressing this area with the thumb and index finger of your other hand. Deeply and firmly make circular motions over this area for 5 minutes. Repeat with your other hand.

▶ See pictures below showing the technique for pressing the Gb20 spot. Find this spot by looking for the depressions at the base of your skull about 2 inches (6 cm) behind your ears. These spots are right in front of the large muscles that run from your head to your neck.

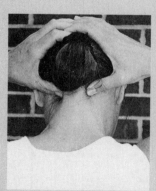 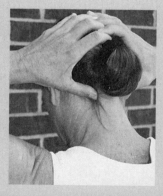

Regulating Sleep

Sleep disturbances trigger headaches for about one in every three migraine sufferers. The *pineal gland* in the brain produces serotonin and converts it into *melatonin*, an important agent for sleep. Both serotonin and melatonin affect pain centers in the brain. Balanced levels of magnesium also influence the pineal gland, with low magnesium linked to both poor sleep and increased headache activity.

Research has shown that headaches become more frequent when people regularly sleep 6 or fewer hours per night on a regular basis. Headaches are also more frequent among people usually sleeping more than 8 hours each night. Therefore, migraine sufferers are encouraged to sleep between 7 and 8 hours each night. Keeping consistent times for going to bed and rising in the morning can also help regulate sleep cycles and improve headaches.

TIPS FOR IMPROVING SLEEP

▶ Practice relaxation techniques at bedtime.

▶ Use your bed only for sleep and sex:
  - Go to bed only when you're sleepy.
  - Don't watch television or read in bed.

▶ Establish and maintain regular sleep and rise times.

▶ Don't nap more than 30 minutes per day.

▶ Reduce evening stimulants (caffeine, nicotine).

▶ Don't drink alcohol before going to bed.

▶ Do aerobic exercise daily, but not right before bedtime.

▶ Make sure the temperature in the bedroom is comfortably cool.

▶ If too much ambient light enters the bedroom, invest in an eye mask.

▶ If noises in the bedroom prevent sleep, try using ear plugs.

▶ If you are unable to fall asleep after 15 minutes, get up and go to another room. Only return to bed when you are sleepy.

It is not unusual for a person with migraines to sleep in on the weekend to try and make up for sleep deprivation during the week, only to find that this provokes a headache. Stick with a more regular sleep schedule by getting up at the same time as on weekdays, going to the bathroom, and eating a small snack before returning to bed. This will help provide a more regular sleep pattern, yet will give you a similar effect as sleeping in on the weekend.

In some cases, sleep is disrupted by *restless leg syndrome* ("jumpy legs") or *sleep apnea*. If you have these or any other sleep disorders that interfere with consistent sleep, talk to your doctor about an evaluation by a sleep specialist. Chronic insomnia must be treated effectively for headaches to be optimally treated. Many times, relaxation methods and sleep hygiene tips are all that are needed. Occasionally, medications are necessary to improve your sleep. Talk to your doctor if you have problems getting to sleep or staying asleep on a regular basis.

Smoking

Nicotine-containing products changes brain levels of a variety of chemicals that influence headache, including endorphins, serotonin, norepinephrine, and dopamine. The ability of nicotine to alter these chemicals explains changes in feelings of anxiety with lighting up and why quitting can be so tough. These chemical changes can also aggravate your headaches. For example, people who smoke are over one-third more likely to develop migraines, compared to non-smokers. Once smokers are having headaches, the use of nicotine products will further lower their headache threshold, making it easier for headaches to occur. Patients sometimes report a reduction in headaches after quitting smoking, although no research studies have confirmed this link.

People interested in quitting smoking can develop a plan and work with a coach for free by contacting 1-800-QUIT-NOW or by visiting http://1800quitnow.cancer.gov, developed by the United States

Department of Health and Human Services, National Institute of Health, and National Cancer Institute.

Diet

Dietary restrictions, such as avoiding foods rich in headache-provoking chemicals, are beneficial for only about one in three migraine sufferers. Most people cannot find food triggers that consistently bring on their headaches. To see if diet influences your headaches, follow a headache restriction diet for 1 month (see pages 77 and 78). If your headaches don't improve during that time, you will have learned that foods are not important triggers for you. If your headaches *do* improve significantly, slowly add foods back into your diet one at a time to identify which foods might be triggering your headaches. In general, a food should trigger a headache within 12 hours of eating it. In some cases, foods only trigger headaches when eaten in large quantities, when consumed in combination with other foods, or when you are also exposed to other triggers. So, for example, you might need to limit caffeine and peanut butter during your menstrual period, but not during the rest of the month.

HEALTHY DIET RECOMMENDATIONS

▶ Eat three meals spaced throughout the day, with healthy snacks in between.

▶ Drink at least ten 8-ounce glasses of water each day:

  • Add more drinks when exercising.

▶ Limit caffeinated beverages to no more than 2 cups or 1 mug each day.

▶ Limit alcohol consumption to a maximum of:

  • 2 drinks per day for an adult man

  • 1 drink per day for an adult woman

  • 1 drink per day for an adult over age 65 years old

Headache Restriction Diet

Food Category	Specific Foods to Avoid
Beverages	Alcohol
	Caffeinated drinks (limit to 2 cups/day)
Breads and cereals	Donuts
	Fresh yeast breads
Dairy	Aged cheeses (bleu, brie, camembert, emmentaler, gouda, gruyere, stilton)
	Buttermilk
	Sour cream
	Yogurt (limit to ½ cup per day)
Fruit	Bananas
	Citrus fruits
	Figs
	Kiwis
	Mangos
	Papaya
	Plums
	Raisins
	Strawberries
Meats	Aged or cured meat (bacon, bologna, pepperoni, salami, sausage)
	Pickled herring
	Snails
Vegetables	Avocados
	Beans
	Corn
	Eggplant
	Olives
	Onions
	Peanuts and peanut butter

	Pickles and pickled food
	Sauerkraut
	Spinach
	Snow peas
	Tomatoes and tomato products
Sweets	Chocolate
Food additives	Aspartame
	Meat tenderizer
	Monosodium glutamate

Headache sufferers are more likely to find that fasting or skipping meals triggers headaches than they are to link a specific food to their headaches. Dehydration is another common headache trigger, so make sure that you consume a sufficient amount of fluids each day.

Devices and Injections Designed to Treat Headaches

Small studies have shown a reduction in headaches from a variety of devices, including:

▶ Night-time mouth splints
▶ Transcranial magnetic stimulation
▶ Injections

Mouth Splints

Jaw muscles, like other muscles in the head and neck, are naturally in balance. When they get out of balance, muscle tightness can occur. Tight and tender jaw muscles can lower the headache threshold. Helping these muscles relax using relaxation techniques and mouth splints can help reduce headache frequency and severity. The Nociceptive Trigeminal Inhibition (NTI) mouth splint has been approved by the Food and Drug Administration (FDA) for the prevention of migraine (www.nti-tss.com). This acrylic mini-splint fits over the front teeth to reduce jaw clenching. In one study, migraine sufferers who also had tenderness of the jaw muscles wore this splint at night and during times of stress. After 2 months, their headache frequency was reduced by two-thirds.

Transcranial Magnetic Stimulation

The back part of the brain is called the *occipital* lobe. Occipital comes from the Latin words *ob* (against) and *capit* (head). This part of the brain controls vision. Research shows that the occipital lobe is more active or *hyperexcitable* in people with migraine. The threshold for activation of migraine is lower in these individuals. Changes in the occipital lobe are often the first changes seen during migraine, so correcting this hyperexcitability may be a way to help raise a person's headache threshold and reduce headache susceptibility.

Transcranial magnetic stimulation provides a weak electrical current by quickly changing magnetic fields. (*Trans* means across and *cranial* means head; so *transcranial* means the current travels across the head.) This electrical current affects brain nerves to help raise the headache threshold. In one study, a hand-held transcranial magnetic stimulation device was placed at the back of the head for 30 seconds during migraine auras. After 2 hours, pain was gone in seven of ten people using the device, compared with five in ten people using an inactive or placebo device. While this is a promising non-drug approach, more study is needed. Transcranial magnetic stimulation devices are not currently available for general use.

Injections

Injecting medications into muscles and nerves around the head and neck can sometimes help reduce headaches. The most effective injections are those that combine a numbing medicine (such as lidocaine or bupivacaine) and a steroid. The numbing medicine temporarily blocks the pain, and the steroid reduces inflammation to help prevent the pain from coming back. The *occipital* nerves leave the neck at the back of the head and then travel over the sides and top of the head. Injections or nerve blocks of these nerves may temporarily help to break a bad headache cycle. The effect of these injections generally lasts days to weeks. You'll get more long-lasting effects if you start neck exercises, relaxation techniques, or other therapies after your headaches have been temporarily reduced by injections.

Botulinum toxin (Botox®) is a muscle-relaxing agent that has been used for decades to cause temporary paralysis to muscles in severe spasm. For example, children with a condition called *torticollis* experience muscle spasms that cause severe and painful twisting of the neck. After the neck muscles have been relaxed with Botox injections, these children can relax their neck muscles. When doctors began using Botox injections of facial muscles to reduce the appearance of wrinkles, they noticed that some people having Botox for wrinkle therapy reported an improvement in their headaches.

Although many large studies have evaluated the possible benefits for migraine sufferers from Botox injections, they have generally shown that Botox injections work no better in reducing headaches than a placebo injection (an injection using no real medicine). For this reason, Botox is generally reserved for headache sufferers for whom strong muscle spasms are a headache trigger. The beneficial effects that might occur with Botox are temporary and should, therefore, be combined with treatments that are more likely to produce long-lasting effects, such as exercises and relaxation therapies. One study recently showed that Botox may be helpful for some people with frequent migraines, so called *chronic migraine* in which headaches occur more often than not (more than 15 days per month).

Manual Therapies

Soothing manual therapies for some pain problems include massage, chiropractic manipulation, and craniosacral therapy. Few research studies have investigated the benefits from these therapies for specifically treating headaches. Those that have been done do not show enough benefit to recommend these treatments for most headache sufferers. Individuals with substantial muscle pain or spasm in addition to headaches, and those with headaches that are consistently triggered by changes in neck posture or using the neck muscles, may get benefit from manual therapies.

MEDICATION TREATMENT OPTIONS

What Really Works?

Most people would prefer not to take any medications for their headaches, but medications are often necessary because migraines are often so disabling. Combining non-drug treatments with medications provides the best option for relieving your headaches while limiting the need for excessive medication use.

Headache medications can be divided into four categories:

- *Acute therapy.* Treats a specific headache episode
- *Prevention therapy.* Reduces the frequency and severity of future headaches
- *Nausea treatments.* Used to reduce severe nausea and vomiting during a headache
- *Rescue therapy.* Taken on those infrequent occasions when other therapies don't work

Acute headache treatments are used to treat infrequent headaches—which occur no more than 2 days per week—and help reduce the pain and other symptoms occurring with a specific headache episode.

Prevention treatments are used to treat frequent headaches—which occur regularly 3 or more days per week—and help reduce future headache frequency and severity. Preventive medications are usually taken on a daily basis.

Take the headache treatment quiz below to determine whether you should focus on acute or acute combined with prevention therapy. In general, acute therapy is used for infrequent headaches—if you regularly get headaches less than 2 days per week, you will likely treat these headaches with acute therapy. If you typically have headaches 3 or more days per week, you will probably need to focus on acute and preventive therapy. Some people use daily prevention therapy (which might include relaxation, stress management, exercises, and/or prevention drugs) plus occasional acute treatment for infrequent severe headaches.

Taking acute medications too frequently can make your headaches more severe and more frequent. This worsening of headaches is called *medication overuse* or *rebound headaches.*

Medication overuse or rebound headaches can develop if short-acting, acute medications are taken more than 2 days per week on a consistent basis. Rebound headaches are easier to prevent than to treat, so see your doctor if you are regularly using acute medications more than 2 days per week.

Make sure you give your acute migraine therapy a good test before deciding it doesn't work. Treat at least three headache episodes and check with your doctor to see if you might need a different dosage

---

SHOULD I CONSIDER USING ACUTE OR PREVENTION THERAPY?

1. Do you usually have a headache for more than 2 days each week?

2. Do you miss school, work, or important social engagements even though you take medications when you have a headache?

3. Do you overuse painkillers to try to prevent headaches from starting?

If you answered "no" to all of these questions, you can probably treat your headaches with acute therapies. If you answered "yes" to any of these questions, talk to your doctor about migraine prevention.

before deciding to try something different. Most drugs work best over a specific dose range, and taking higher doses generally won't give you any better effect than using the recommended effective dose. You will, however, get more unwanted side effects at higher doses.

Effective Over-the-Counter Remedies

Over-the-counter analgesics or pain-relieving medications include aspirin and nonsteroidal anti-inflammatory drugs (NSAIDs), such as ibuprofen (Advil®, Motrin®), naproxen (Naprosyn®, Aleve®), and acetaminophen (Tylenol®).

In general, aspirin and NSAIDs are more effective for relieving headaches than is acetaminophen. Side effects are more common with aspirin, ibuprofen, and naproxen, especially stomach upset, bleeding, and dizziness. Many people use acetaminophen because they tolerate it better than aspirin, ibuprofen, or naproxen. People with a history of bleeding problems or stomach ulcers generally use acetaminophen. None of these pain-relieving medications should be used more than 2 days per week on average, to avoid medication overuse or rebound headaches. Overuse can also damage your kidneys and liver.

Caffeine is frequently added to over-the-counter headache remedies because it increases the *analgesic* (pain-killing) effect of these remedies. Research shows that adding 100 milligrams of caffeine to a nonsteroidal anti-inflammatory medication increases the number of people who obtain migraine relief by one and one-half times! Caffeine is included in over-the-counter analgesics such as Excedrin® (65 milligrams caffeine per tablet) and Anacin® (32 milligrams caffeine per tablet). If you don't have an analgesic-plus-caffeine medication at home, you can add caffeine yourself by taking your over-the-counter analgesic with a caffeinated beverage. The amounts of caffeine in common beverages are:

▶ 7 ounces of coffee has 65 to 135 milligrams.

▶ 7 ounces of tea has 40 to 60 milligrams.

▶ 12 ounces of cola has 30 to 50 milligrams.

Be aware that some researchers believe excessive caffeine use (more than two cups of coffee daily) may lead to headache worsening or rebound headaches.

TIPS FOR EFFECTIVE USE OF OVER-THE-COUNTER MEDICATIONS

▶ Aspirin, ibuprofen, and naproxen are generally more effective than acetaminophen.

▶ Use acetaminophen if you don't tolerate the other analgesics.

▶ Use acetaminophen if you have a bleeding disorder or gastric ulcers.

▶ Add caffeine to analgesics to improve pain relief.

▶ Limit over-the-counter drugs to no more than 2 days per week.

▶ Let your doctor know about all over-the-counter drugs you use.

Prescription Drugs

Prescription NSAIDs can also be used to effectively treat migraine. An effervescent formulation of the anti-inflammatory drug diclofenac (Cambia®) was recently approved as a specific migraine therapy. Prescription-strength ibuprofen and naproxen contain higher doses than those available as over-the-counter medications. For example, three over-the-counter ibuprofen tablets of 200 mg each equals one 600-mg prescription ibuprofen tablet.

Other prescription painkillers, such as opioid or narcotic medications, are generally ineffective against migraine symptoms. Opioids are best used as rescue treatments when other, more typically effective therapies have failed to help. The barbiturate (sedative) drug *butalbital* (Fiorinal®, Fioricet®) has not been shown to reduce migraines and frequently results in overuse and rebound headaches, and should generally be avoided.

The year 1993 ushered in a new era of headache treatment with the release of *sumatriptan* (Imitrex®). This medication revolutionized the treatment of migraine. Subsequently, six more medications similar to sumatriptan, called *triptans*, were released. As of January 2010, suma-triptan became available as a generic medication and has significantly dropped in price compared to the other triptans, which are available as brand name only. The triptans are generally quite effective and very well tolerated, especially if taken early in an attack. There are several differ-ences among the individual triptan therapies, with some providing more rapid onset of relief and others having fewer side effects. Four in five migraine sufferers obtain relief from a triptan. If one doesn't work, be sure to try a least two others before deciding that triptans don't work for you.

Dihydroergotamine (DHE®, Migranal®), with an action similar to the triptans, is another medication specifically designed to treat migraines. In general, however, triptans are more effective than DHE, with fewer side effects. DHE generally lasts longer than any of the triptans.

Adding an NSAID, such as naproxen, to a triptan can help increase headache reduction and prolong the pain-relieving effect. A combination of naproxen plus sumatriptan is now available combined into one tablet (Treximet®). By combining two different ways to treat a migraine episode, this combination is more effective than either of its two component parts alone.

Anti-nausea drugs, or *anti-emetics*, may be helpful to add to anal-gesics or other acute headache treatment when nausea is a major prob-lem. Aggressive treatment of nausea may be critical to the success of your treatment program, because anti-nausea therapy can also improve stomach emptying. During a migraine episode, and even when you're not having a migraine, stomach emptying is slower in people with migraine. This condition, called *gastroparesis*, causes recently consumed food, stomach juices, and medications to remain in the stomach. This

TRIPTANS

Triptan	Typical Dosage	Advantages
Fastest Acting		
Sumatriptan (Imitrex®)	6 mg injection 20 mg nasal spray	Relief may begin after 10–15 minutes. Best and fastest results occur with injection. Nasal spray provides faster relief than using sumatriptan tablets.
Zolmitriptan (Zomig®)	5 mg nasal spray	Relief may begin after 10 minutes.
Fast Acting		
Almotriptan (Axert®)	12.5 mg tablet	Relief after about 45–60 minutes. Well tolerated.
Eletriptan (Relpax®)	40–80 mg tablet	Relief after about 30 minutes. Very effective.
Rizatriptan (Maxalt®)	10 mg tablet	Relief after about 30 minutes. Very effective. Tablet that dissolves in the mouth is available for added convenience.
Sumatriptan (Imitrex®)	50–100 mg tablet	Relief after about 45–60 minutes.
Zolmitriptan (Zomig®)	5 mg tablet	Relief after about 45–60 minutes. Tablet that dissolves in the mouth is available for added convenience.
Slower Acting		
Frovatriptan (Frova®)	2.5 mg tablet	Relief may take up to 4 hours to start. Sustained effect, but efficacy is relatively low. Few side effects.
Naratriptan (Amerge®)	2.5 mg tablet	Relief may take up to 4 hours to start. Sustained effect, but efficacy is relatively low. Few side effects.

can worsen your nausea and make your medications work more slowly, because it takes longer for the medications to get into your system. For this reason, the anti-nausea drug *metoclopramide* (Reglan®), which also helps speed stomach emptying, can reduce nausea and help your other migraine drugs work better and faster.

If your usual acute treatments don't work for a particular headache, you might need a rescue therapy. Many medications can be used for rescue. Some of the more common ones are: *chlorpromazine* (Thorazine®); a combination of *isometheptene mucate, dichloral-*

ANTI-NAUSEA MEDICATIONS

Nausea Treatment	Typical Adult Dosage	Common Side Effects
Domperidone (Motilium®; not available in the United States)	20–30 mg tablet	Dizziness, dry mouth, nervousness
Prochlorperazine (Compazine®)	10 mg tablet 25 mg rectal suppository	Constipation, dizziness, sleepiness, dry mouth, restlessness
Promethazine (Phenergan®)	25 mg tablet 12.5–25 mg rectal suppository	Sleepiness, dizziness, restlessness, palpitations
Metoclopramide (Reglan®)	10 mg tablet or intramuscular injection, or 20 mg rectal suppository	Sleepiness, restlessness, anxiety, insomnia, depression
Ondansetron (Zofran®)	5 mL oral solution or 4 mg tablet or orally disintegrating tablet you can take without water	Blurred vision, diarrhea, constipation, dizziness, fatigue. Usually very well tolerated.
Trimethobenzamide (Tigan®)	100–300 mg capsule	Diarrhea, dizziness, sleepiness, blurred vision

phenazone, and *acetaminophen* (Midrin®); and *hydroxyzine* (Vistaril®). Opioid pain medications are often not helpful, and should be used sparingly because of a higher risk for developing rebound headaches relative to other medications.

What Medications Help Prevent Headaches?

All of the drugs used as migraine prevention therapy were originally designed to treat some other health condition, such as high blood pressure, mood disorders, or epilepsy. When these drugs were used in large numbers of people with these other conditions, patients and doctors began to notice headache improvement. Many of these drugs have now been tested in large research studies to prove that they are also effective for preventing chronic headaches. Among the antidepressants, the older tricyclic antidepressants such as amitriptyline and *imipramine* (Tofranil®) are considerably more effective than the newer classes of antidepressants and anti-anxiety agents (such as the selective serotonin reuptake inhibitors [SSRIs] or serotonin noradrenergic reuptake inhibitors [SNRIs]).

Remember—prevention medications usually take several months to take effect, and they probably will not totally eliminate all future headaches. In general, doctors consider a prevention therapy to be successful if the number of headaches you have decreases by about half after using a prevention treatment for 3 months.

How Can Alternative Drug Formulations Help?

Although most people prefer to take medications by mouth, drug absorption is often limited by poor absorption from the stomach and gastroparesis. During a migraine attack, it takes over 10 percent longer for the stomach contents to empty. This means that your body will have a lesser amount of drug available, and it will take longer for that drug to reach target organs during a migraine attack. Because gastroparesis

PREVENTION MEDICATIONS

Headache Prevention Drug	Typical Adult Dose	Common Side Effects
Most Effective Drugs for Migraine Prevention		
Beta-blocker blood pressure medications	Propranolol (Inderal®) 80–160 mg long-acting form daily Timolol (Blocadren®) 20 mg daily	Avoid if you have diabetes, asthma, or slow heart rate
Antidepressants	Tricyclics are the most effective antidepressant class for headache prevention; e.g., amitriptyline (Elavil®) or imipramine (Tofranil®) 25–100 mg, 2 hours before bed	Dry mouth, dizziness, constipation, sleepiness, weight gain
Anti-seizure drugs	Divalproex sodium (Depakote®) 125–250 mg twice daily Topiramate (Topamax®) 50 mg twice daily	Sleepiness, weight gain, hair loss, bleeding problems, menstrual irregularities with divalproex. Word-finding difficulty, numbness and tingling of extremities, weight loss, and sedation with topiramate. *Divalproex should not be used if there is any chance of pregnancy.*
Moderately Effective Drugs for Migraine Prevention		
Other anti-seizure drugs	Gabapentin (Neurontin®) 100–400 mg, two to three times daily Pregabalin (Lyrica®) 50–100 mg, two to three times daily	Dizziness or clumsiness, sleepiness, double vision, changes in bowel habits or nausea, swelling

PREVENTION MEDICATIONS (CONTINUED)

Headache Prevention Drug	Typical Adult Dose	Common Side Effects
Other anti-seizure drugs	Levetiracetam (Keppra®) 500 mg twice daily. Lamotrigine (Lamictal®) 50 mg twice daily	
Calcium-channel blocker blood pressure medications	Flunarizine 5–10 mg daily (Sibelium®; not available in the United States, but more effective than verapamil) Verapamil (Calan®, Isoptin®) 240–480 mg long-acting form daily	Constipation, dizziness, nausea, low blood pressure, mood changes, insomnia, fatigue

Sometimes Used for Migraine Prevention

Antihistamine	Cinnarizine 25 mg three times daily or 75 mg at bedtime (Stugeron®; not available in North America). Cyproheptadine (Periactin®) 4 mg, two to three times daily	Sleepiness, dizziness, blurred vision, stomach upset or bowel problems, weight gain, dry nose and mouth
Some muscle relaxers	Tizanidine (Zanaflex®) 2–8 mg, two to three times daily Cyclobenzaprine (Flexeril®) 10 mg, three times daily Orphenadrine (Norflex®) 100 mg twice daily	Constipation, dizziness, sleepiness, dry mouth, weakness

PREVENTION MEDICATIONS (CONTINUED)

Headache Prevention Drug	Typical Adult Dose	Common Side Effects
Angiotensin blocker blood pressure medications	Candesartan (Atacand®) 4–16 mg daily Lisinopril (Zestril®, Prinivil®) 10–20 mg daily	Dizziness, blurred vision, sore throat, nausea, runny or stuffy nose, low blood pressure, cough

limits the effectiveness of many migraine pills, drug manufacturers are developing and testing alternative migraine therapies. Drugs given using alternative routes of administration are called different *formulations*. The advantages of taking a medication using a different formulation can be:

▶ A more consistent response
▶ Quicker onset of effectiveness
▶ More effective
▶ Less likelihood of the same migraine returning
▶ Fewer side effects

New medication development is an exciting and active area of research. The table on page 92 lists medications designed with new formulations that may be helpful for migraine sufferers.

NUTRITIONAL PRODUCTS AND SUPPLEMENTS

Which natural therapies really work? Cutting through the hype on natural therapies for migraine can be confusing. When evaluating nutritional products and supplements for possible use in migraine treatment, your doctor should be your first source for unbiased, expert information.

NEW FORMULATIONS OF MIGRAINE DRUGS

Formulation Route	Advantages	Examples
Needle-free injections	Compressed nitrogen gas forces liquid drug into subcutaneous tissues, providing rapid drug delivery to cells without a needle for injection. Peak drug levels achieved 2 minutes faster than with traditional injection with a needle.	*Sumavel DosePro™ (sumatriptan)
Inhaled drug	Lungs provide a large area from which drugs can be rapidly absorbed, with direct access to the blood.	*Levadex™ (dihydroergotamine) Staccato® prochlorperazine (aerosol prochlorperazine)
Intranasal	Affects activation of migraine pain fibers that travel through the nasal passages. May provide rapid pain relief with few side effects.	Intranasal carbon dioxide Intranasal ketorolac Intranasal sumatriptan powder
Transdermal	Most drugs cannot be reliably absorbed through the skin. Drugs are more consistently absorbed by using a low electrical current in a patch, called *iontophoresis*. Absorption can also be improved by inserting drugs into tiny vesicles, called *elastic liposomes*. Elastic liposomes can easily change their shape, making it easier for them to squeeze through pores	Zelrix™ (sumatriptan iontophoresis patch) Diclofenac elastic liposome Rizatriptan elastic liposome

NEW FORMULATIONS OF MIGRAINE DRUGS

Formulation Route	Advantages	Examples
	and into the skin. Transdermal drugs often work quickly and provide good long-lasting relief.	
Transmucosal	Drug is sprayed over the tongue, called *lingual*. Rapid absorption within the mouth avoids problems with absorption through the stomach during a migraine.	Sumatriptan lingual spray
Oral drug	Effervescent powder provides more rapid and complete absorption than with traditional pills. Pain relief starts after 15 minutes with effervescent powder versus 60 minutes with the same drug in a tablet.	*Cambia™ (diclofenac)

Drugs that are currently approved for migraine and available are marked with an asterisk (*).

Vitamins

Riboflavin

The normal daily recommended amount of riboflavin for general health in adults is 1–2 mg. This amount would be found in about 2 cups of milk or yogurt. High-dose riboflavin (400 mg of riboflavin daily for 3 months) has been shown to reduce the number of migraine attacks by half. Effective doses for children and adolescents are 200–400 mg daily. Most pharmacies don't carry the 400-mg tablet, and you may have to ask your pharmacist to order it. Riboflavin is generally very well tolerated. And don't worry about overdosing—riboflavin is a water-soluble vitamin, and your body will take what it needs and excrete the rest, so it can't build up to toxic levels.

Coenzyme Q10

Also called *ubiquinone* and *CoQ10*, this coenzyme is made by the body and can also be obtained by eating meats and seafood. Coenzyme Q10 100 mg three times daily or 150 mg once daily for 3 months reduces migraine frequency by up to one-half. Improvement is better with the 150-mg daily dose; both doses are well tolerated with very few side effects. Taking 200 mg twice daily is helpful for some people with migraine-related problems. Coenzyme Q10 can affect blood sugar metabolism and may change blood clotting, so don't use CoQ10 if you have diabetes or bleeding disorders, or are using blood thinners.

Minerals

Magnesium

Magnesium levels in the blood are often low in people with migraines. Daily adult requirements of magnesium for good health are 300–400 mg, an amount that you could obtain by eating 2 to 3 ounces of roasted pumpkin seeds or three to four bowls of bran cereal daily. Some people with normal blood levels of magnesium have low brain magnesium levels, so a blood test may not necessarily tell you if magnesium might be helpful for you. Taking a 600-mg magnesium supplement for adults or lower doses in children reduces migraine frequency by about one-third. Another preparation you might try is magnesium oxide, 400 mg daily. Some people find that the slow release preparation, Slow Mag or Mag Delay, are better tolerated.

Herbs

Butterbur (Petasites hybridus)

This is a perennial shrub. Its root extract reduces inflammation and is used to treat asthma and migraine. Butterbur is the most effective nutritional remedy for migraines. Doses of 50–75 mg twice daily have been shown to reduce headaches by up to one-half after about 3 months. Children may use 25 mg twice daily. Most people complain of few side effects when taking butterbur, although about one in four will experience digestive system complaints, most commonly burping. It can be ordered online at www.migraineaid.com.

Feverfew (Tanacetum parthenium L.)

Feverfew comes from a flower that looks like a daisy. Its main active ingredient is *parthenolide*. Feverfew reduces inflammation and—as its name suggests—it is commonly used to treat fevers, arthritis, menstrual discomfort, and migraines. Migraine frequency decreases by one-fourth in some people taking about 100 mg of feverfew daily. Parthenolide content varies widely among different brands of feverfew, and a preparation must contain at least 0.2 percent parthenolide to prevent migraines. A higher amount of parthenolide (0.5 percent) is available in feverfew manufactured in Israel (available at Galilee Herbal Remedies). This higher concentration may be more beneficial for reducing migraines. Feverfew decreases clotting and should be avoided if you have a bleeding disorders or use aspirin, anti-inflammatory medications, or other medications that decrease clotting.

Peppermint Oil

This oil is derived from the plant *Mentha piperita*, with the main active components being menthol and menthon. Peppermint reduces gastric distress and acts as a topical analgesic. A solution of 10 g peppermint oil in alcohol may be applied lightly to the forehead and temples during a headache attack, and repeated after 15 and 30 minutes. In one study, migraine improved by at least half in 58 percent of people treating their migraine with topical peppermint oil compared with only 17 percent using an inactive placebo. Migraine pain was completely eliminated for 38 percent treating with topical peppermint oil compared with only 12 percent using the placebo. Although not specifically tested for other headaches, topical peppermint oil may also be worth trying during a migraine attack. It should never be applied to or near the faces of infants or small children, as this may result in serious and potentially life-threatening spasm of respiratory structures and respiratory distress.

RECOMMENDED DOSES OF NUTRITIONAL PRODUCTS FOR HEADACHE

▶ During a headache attack:

- Topical peppermint oil: 10 g peppermint oil in alcohol applied to forehead and temples during a headache

▶ For prevention treatment:

- Minerals and vitamins:

  – Magnesium: 600 mg daily

  – Riboflavin: 400 mg daily

  – Coenzyme Q10: 150 mg daily

- Herbs:

  – Butterbur: 50 to 100 mg twice daily

  – Feverfew: 100 mg of feverfew containing 0.2 percent parthenolide daily

- Sleep hormone:

  – Melatonin 3 mg taken 30 minutes before bed

Hormones

Melatonin

In one study, the sleep hormone melatonin in a dose of 3 mg taken 30 minutes before bedtime for 3 months reduced the number of migraines by almost two-thirds and reduced migraine severity by half. A few people taking melatonin reported side effects of excessive sleepiness, hair loss, and increased sexual libido.

PUTTING TOGETHER A TREATMENT PLAN

Creating a Personal Strategy for Your Migraines

You can maximize the likelihood that your headache will be controlled by combining effective medication and non-medication options. Initial

COMPLEMENTARY TREATMENTS FOR HEADACHE

Effective	Moderately Effective	Ineffective
Biofeedback	Feverfew (*Tanacetum*	Acupuncture
Butterbur (*Petasites*)	*parthenium*)	Botulinum toxin
Relaxation	Coenzyme Q10	injections
Stress management	Diet	
	Exercise	
	Intraoral appliance	
	Magnesium	
	Melatonin	
	Physical therapy	
	Riboflavin	
	Sleep hygiene	
	Smoking cessation	

treatment selections should include those therapies that have been proven most effective in most people. Treatments that have been shown to be less effective for migraine, such as acupuncture or botulinum toxin injections, will generally not be helpful, unless you have significant muscle tightness.

Recording Headaches in Daily Diaries

Why Should I Keep Track of My Headaches?

Patients are often surprised when they begin tracking their headaches. They often find that their headaches are actually more frequent and disabling than they had thought. It can be a real eye-opener to count up the days you missed from school, work, or family activities, and then add in those additional days that you were much less productive because of headaches.

GENERAL PRINCIPLES OF EFFECTIVE MIGRAINE MANAGEMENT

▶ Use a headache diary to keep track of your headache pattern, what triggers your headaches, and how well your treatments are working.

▶ Include non-medication treatments.

▶ Focus on prevention therapies if your headaches typically occur more than a few days each week.

▶ Treat individual headache episodes early, while symptoms are still mild. Don't postpone treatment until symptoms are severe and more difficult to treat.

▶ Use a stepwise approach to treat individual headache episodes. Mild headaches often improve with over-the-counter NSAIDs. Use more aggressive treatments, such as a triptan medication, if your headache is more severe.

▶ Treat nausea early and aggressively.

▶ Have a rescue plan in place to prevent the need for emergency room or urgent care visits for headache.

▶ Talk to your healthcare provider about changing your treatments if you:

- Typically have headaches 2 or more days per week

- Frequently use rescue medications

- Have significant disability associated with your headaches

- End up going to the ER or Urgent Care Clinic for headache treatment

▶ Only use medications prescribed for you, and *never* use a medication prescribed for another person, whether for migraine or another condition.

Diaries can help show you headache patterns and whether your treatments are working or not. Recording headache severity several times daily will give you a more complete picture of your headache pattern than using a once-daily severity recording. Be sure to bring your calendar to every visit with your healthcare provider to help determine what's happening with your headaches.

DAILY HEADACHE DIARY

Day	Migraine severity				Possible triggers		Treatments
	None	Mild	Moderate	Severe	Drugs	Non-drugs	
Sunday							
Morning							
Noon							
Bedtime							
Monday							
Morning							
Noon							
Evening							
Bedtime							
Tuesday							
Morning							
Noon							
Evening							
Bedtime							

Daily Headache Diary (CONTINUED)

Day	Migraine severity				Possible triggers		Treatments
	None	Mild	Moderate	Severe	Drugs	Non-drugs	
Wednesday							
Morning							
Noon							
Evening							
Bedtime							
Thursday							
Morning							
Noon							
Evening							
Bedtime							
Friday							
Morning							
Noon							

Daily Headache Diary (CONTINUED)

Day	Migraine severity				Possible triggers		Treatments
	None	Mild	Moderate	Severe	Drugs	Non-drugs	
Evening							
Bedtime							
Saturday							
Morning							
Noon							
Evening							
Bedtime							

Diary instructions. Record headache severity four times daily—even on days when you don't have a headache. Note the occurrence of possible common triggers each day—such as stress, poor sleep, and skipping meals. Record the date of your menstrual period under the trigger column. List all over-the-counter, prescription, and non-drug treatments you use with each headache. Review this diary with your healthcare provider on a regular basis.

Migraine Treatment Assessment Strategies: Tracking Your Progress and Response to Treatment

Well-known headache expert Dr. Richard Lipton recently developed the five-question Migraine Treatment Optimization Questionnaire to determine whether an individual's migraine treatment is working well, as shown below. If you answer "no" to any of the first three questions, you may need to treat your migraine earlier, adjust medication doses, or change treatments. If you answer "yes" to all of the questions except the last one, you may wish to add more non-drug therapies to your treatment regimen.

MIGRAINE TREATMENT OPTIMIZATION QUESTIONNAIRE

Answer the following questions based on your headaches over the last 4 weeks:

1. Can you quickly return to normal activities after taking your migraine medication?

2. Can you usually count on your migraine medication to relieve pain within 2 hours?

3. Does one dose of medication usually relieve your headache and keep it away for at least 24 hours?

4. Do you have problems with side effects from your migraine medication?

5. Are you comfortable enough with your medication to plan your daily activities?

If your migraine treatment is working well, you will have answered "yes" to all of these questions. If you answered "no" to any of them, take this quiz with you to your doctor to talk about ways to improve your treatment.

Practice Logs for Non-Drug Treatments

Relaxation Exercise Log	Morning Relaxation			Evening Relaxation		
	Time (minutes)	Tension before	Tension after	Time (minutes)	Tension before	Tension after
Sunday						
Monday						
Tuesday						
Wednesday						
Thursday						
Friday						
Saturday						

When you are first learning relaxation techniques, practice them twice daily for 15–20 minutes for each practice session. Practice in a quiet environment. Record actual time spent for each session. Rate and log tension as none (0), mild (1), moderate (2), or severe (3).

STRETCHING EXERCISE LOG

	Morning Stretches			Evening Stretches		
	Time (minutes)	Pain before	Pain after	Time (minutes)	Pain before	Pain after
Sunday						
Monday						
Tuesday						
Wednesday						
Thursday						
Friday						
Saturday						

Stretching exercises should be done twice daily for 15–20 minutes in each exercise session. Stretching should be completed at least 4 days per week. Do stretches in front of the television or with music playing to reduce boredom. Log the time spent stretching, as well as your pain levels before and after exercise. Rate and log pain as none (0), mild (1), moderate (2), or severe (3).

AEROBIC EXERCISE WALKING LOG

Research has shown that you get good health benefits from walking 150 minutes per week. You'll actually get better health benefits if you break your walks into several short walks rather than doing a few long aerobic exercise sessions. To see if you achieve this goal, log each time you briskly walk for at least 10 minutes. Check off one box for each 10 minutes you walk. You'll have reached your target when you check off 15 boxes each week. As you get into better shape, you can increase your walking pace to increase your total distance.

Day	10-minutes of walking (put a check in a box for every 10 minutes you walk each day, up to a maximum of 40 minutes per day)			
	10 minutes	10 minutes	10 minutes	10 minutes
Sunday				
Monday				
Tuesday				
Wednesday				
Thursday				
Friday				
Saturday				

Total number of boxes per week: _____ (number should be at least 15)

SUMMARY

▶ Headache treatments can be divided into acute, prevention, anti-nausea, and rescue therapies.

▶ If your headaches typically occur more than 2 days each week, you'll need to consider preventive treatments in addition to the acute treatments.

▶ Effective non-drug treatments include relaxation, stress management, exercises, acupressure, and healthy lifestyle changes.

▶ The most effective medications for treating an individual headache episode are over-the-counter analgesics with caffeine, NSAIDs, and triptan drugs.

▶ Effective headache prevention therapies include medications, nutritional therapies, and non-drug treatments.

▶ Recording headache activities every day in a diary can provide valuable information about your headache pattern that can help direct treatment selection. Diaries also help identify whether your treatments are working.

4

Controlling Migraine During Childhood and Adolescence

Headaches are relatively common in children, and migraine is the most common type of chronic headache they experience. Many children assume that having headaches is a normal part of life, especially when they have family members who also get them. For this reason, childhood headaches are sometimes not recognized until they begin to interfere with school. Although headaches can occur even in very young children, they occur most commonly in young people between 12 and 15 years old. In young children, headaches are actually more common in boys. Once puberty starts, headaches become much more common in girls.

Research studies have shown that many youngsters occasionally get headaches, with frequent headaches occurring in a sizable number. In a recent survey of over 1,000 adolescents ages 12–15, two in every three reported getting headaches at least occasionally. One in every three youngsters had a headache at least once a month, and one in five reported having a headache at least once a week!

Note that, in this chapter, we are using the terms "daughter," "her," and "she," referring to girls, since this is a book primarily about women and girls, but all of the information applies equally to boys.

Headaches differ in boys and girls:

▶ In early childhood, about 5 percent of boys and girls have migraines.
▶ Migraines start at a younger age in boys—typically around age 5.
▶ Migraines in girls usually start later—typically around puberty, with age 12 the most common age for migraines to start in girls.
▶ Migraines often disappear as boys reach adulthood, but they continue throughout adulthood in girls.
▶ Individual migraine episodes are generally more frequent and last longer in girls.

Childhood headaches are also different from adult headaches. Most importantly, headache episodes in young people tend to be shorter in duration, with migraines usually lasting only 1–2 hours before resolving. They are often associated with abdominal pain, involve less nausea than in adults, and are often relieved by sleep. Younger children often have a difficult time describing their headache symptoms, so it may be helpful to have them draw a picture of what their headache feels like to better understand what symptoms they are experiencing. Having your child keep a headache diary is also helpful to evaluate headache frequency and treatment success. Remember—this is her diary and needs to be completed by her and not you! Very young children might have an easier time using a smiley face scale.

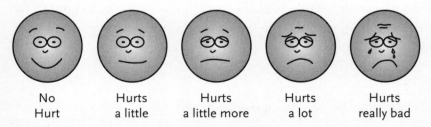

| No | Hurts | Hurts | Hurts | Hurts |
| Hurt | a little | a little more | a lot | really bad |

Which face shows what your headache feels like?

Headache Management During School

Will Migraines Keep Your Child from Making the Grade?

Childhood headache is important because children with headaches miss school about twice as often as other children. One study found that the average child without headaches was absent about 3½ days during the school year, compared with almost 8 days for the average child with headaches.

Missing school because of headaches can be a very difficult issue. Occasional absences can quickly deteriorate into a downward cycle, ending with excessive absences, falling behind, and increased stress. Sometimes parents are forced to consider homebound education.

Homebound education should not be confused with home schooling, where the parent has opted to provide full educational training in the home environment. Homebound education is provided by the child's school after a substantial number of absences. In many cases, homebound materials provide modified and abbreviated training for core classes only, with a minimal number of hours weekly required for educational instruction, rather than the full training provided in

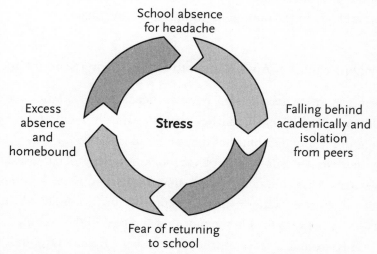

School absence increases a student's stress. Missing school for headaches worsens stress levels, which further aggravates headaches.

school. The goal of homebound education is to prevent the child from falling too far behind academically, so that she can successfully re-enter the classroom when she is able to return to school. The longer the child remains on homebound education, the more difficult this transition back to school will be. One of the goals of headache treatment in school-age children is to keep them in school. Homebound learning should only be considered as a very last resort.

Successful management of disabling headaches often requires a team approach involving the child's teacher, school nurse, school psychologist, healthcare provider, parents, and—most of all—the child. Everyone involved must be in agreement and have the same goals in mind. This can often be quite challenging for parents, because adopting a firm, but fair stance while feeling empathy for the child can be difficult. Although it's hard to send your child off to school when she tells you she's having a headache, regular attendance in school is one of the best ways to keep her symptoms from actually getting worse. A formal, individualized written treatment plan (using the material in this chapter) with plans for both treating and preventing headaches should be developed with your healthcare provider. Make sure this plan is distributed to the school and that everyone—you, your child, your doctor, and the school—have the same goals for headache treatment.

Why Do Headaches Always Seem to Occur During School Hours?

There is a strong relationship between headaches and school stress. Children with chronic headaches characteristically report head pain during the school day, but that they are headache-free for after-school activities, weekends, and school vacations. A survey of almost 2,000 adolescents with migraine found that headaches most commonly occurred during school hours, typically on Monday through Wednesday between 6:00 in the morning and 6:00 in the evening.

This strong influence of school stress on migraine in children and adolescents frequently causes parents, teachers, and fellow students to

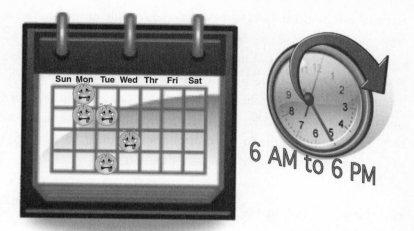

Migraines in children and adolescents most commonly occur Mondays, Tuesdays, and Wednesdays between 6:00 in the morning and 6:00 in the evening.

question whether headaches are real or just a convenient excuse to avoid schoolwork. As your child's parent and strongest advocate, it's important to understand that this link between school and migraine reflects the high stress impact that school has on headaches. Just because headaches usually occur during school hours doesn't mean that your child is making them up.

Stress is a major trigger for headaches in both children and adults. Because children's lives are centered around school, their stresses typically occur there. These stresses can be related to academics, social relationships, scheduling problems, and other difficulties. When you're an adult, you don't treat work stresses that might be triggering headaches by quitting work. In the same way, children whose headaches occur more at school shouldn't stop attending school. Rather, stress management training should be personalized to target the academic and social issues that are likely to be triggering headaches. School avoidance actu-

Migraines in youngsters most commonly occur during school hours. Research shows that most migraines occur during the school year on a Monday, Tuesday, or Wednesday, and between 6 a.m. and 6 p.m.

ally adds additional stresses to children—both academic difficulties and social problems caused by isolation from peers.

Your child needs to understand that her "job" is attending school and, unless the headache is so severe that she is vomiting, the child should attend school—even on days when she has a headache. Luckily, most headaches in children and adolescents only last a few hours, so if they do miss some time in the morning, they should be returned to school as soon as possible to minimize time lost.

How Should I Talk to My Daughter About Migraines?

Be sure to discuss migraines openly with your child. Let her know that migraines are a real medical problem caused by imbalances in pain chemicals in the brain. If other family members have migraine, let your child know that people usually inherit a susceptibility for migraines. It's important for your child to know that these headaches are real and not caused by something she did or didn't do. It's equally important to let her know that migraines are treatable and that you expect that they can be brought under control by using a variety of treatments. If *you* have migraines, make sure you're doing a good job of taking care of your own headaches and incorporating effective non-drug treatments into your daily routine to provide a good role model for your youngster.

When Will the Headaches Go Away, So My Child Can Get Back to a Normal Life?

Don't expect that headaches will improve until your child returns to a more normal lifestyle. Neither the parents nor the young person can expect that migraines will go away *before* returning to a regular routine.

Involvement in regular activities keeps the brain and nervous system busy and distracts it. Lack of activity allows teenagers to focus all of their attention on their headaches, which, in turn, increases the severity of their pain. The first step in headache management is not getting rid of the pain, but getting rid of the misery that headaches produce. Following a regular routine is necessary. Function improves first—pain improves later. When your child is home sick from school, she may feel miserable because of headache symptoms, but also because of missing interacting with friends, concerns about falling behind in schoolwork, and poor self-image. The longer she stays at home, the worse this misery becomes.

When your child is at school, walking between classes, sitting at a desk, listening to the teacher, and chatting with friends all provide important distractions for her brain. Walking may not seem very interesting intellectually, but it is very exciting for the brain and nervous system. Muscles and joints are moving at different rates, balance must be maintained, body temperature must be regulated, the eyes view the environment, and the child's mind may focus on a friend's conversation. These activities take energy and attention away and provide a distraction from the pain and misery of headache.

How Do We Get Back to a More Normal Life?

Your youngster needs to resume a more regular routine, with school at the center. School attendance must be a top priority for both child and family. Even when your child states a preference to remain home with a headache, you need to insist on school attendance as the primary target of headache therapy. School is important to social and emotional development in addition to intellectual development. Homebound education cannot equal the experience of the classroom.

Establish a normal daily routine for your daughter:

▶ *Maintain a regular bedtime.* Bedtime needs to be no later than 10 p.m. If your child is unable to sleep, allow her to listen to the radio or read a book. She should not watch television, text friends, or snack after bedtime.

▶ *Maintain a regular rising time.* This needs to allow adequate time to get ready for school. Regular bed and rising times need to be maintained, even for kids who are already out of school on homebound education.

▶ *Maintain regular meal times.* Children need to eat breakfast, lunch, and dinner every day. Family meal time is an important time to share news of the day's events and problems, and also learn how other family members handle their stresses and resolve conflicts.

▶ *Maintain a regular homework time and location*, not in front of the television or computer games. Scheduling homework time helps to prevent the amount of homework that needs doing from building up, which adds more stress.

▶ *Maintain enjoyable leisure activities.* Fun activities will ideally take your child out of the house and encourage socialization. Limit the time spent playing computer games, surfing the Internet, and watching television or movies. Encourage activities such as walking, sports, shopping, and socializing.

What If My Child Is Already Receiving Homebound Education?

Work with your child's teachers and guidance counselor to get her back into the classroom as soon as possible. If your youngster has been receiving homebound education long-term, the initial focus needs to be on resuming a normal home routine before returning to the classroom. Within a few weeks, return to school must follow, beginning with a gradual reentry if possible. Initially, your child should return to school to attend courses in which she has the most confidence, as well as lunch. If it is not possible to return to school part-time, then she will need to return full-time. Stick with your plan for returning to school, even if your child insists on coming home during the day the first few days after returning. If the attempt to return is not successful, talk to the school counselor about additional issues that may be causing your child's inability to reenter school.

Once back at school, your child should be allowed to leave the classroom to go to the nurse, if needed. Unless she is vomiting, however, she should be returned to the classroom after 15–20 minutes. At the nurse's office, the child may use some of those non-medication treatment techniques described below, as well as medications prescribed for treating the headaches.

What's My Role as a Parent?

Your job as parent is *not* to get rid of your child's headache symptoms! Don't expect that you can make the pain go away. Pampering your child will not improve her headaches. Your job is to ensure that your child gets up, dressed, and to school every day unless she is vomiting.

Your other important job is to help reinforce and encourage normal childhood activities. Every youngster should have a good self-identity that does not center around being a patient or a headache sufferer. Your adolescent, for example, might see herself as a tenth grader, violinist, athlete, good

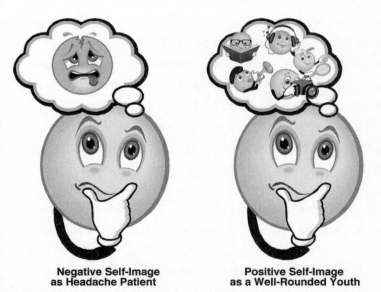

**Negative Self-Image
as Headache Patient**

**Positive Self-Image
as a Well-Rounded Youth**

Encourage your child to develop a healthy, positive self-image rather than focusing excessively on headaches.

student, scout, or avid shopper, rather than as a headache patient. The headache should not be a significant part of your adolescent's identity.

Parents play a critical role in the success of the treatment plan. You need to be a firm, but fair advocate for your child. You must help your child without enabling negative behaviors. Parents need to reinforce their children's treatment strategy, encourage school attendance, monitor compliance with medications and non-drug treatment recommendations, and educate school staff about the child's needs. Parents also must be vigilant to avoid overcommitment by the child, because participating in too many activities in addition to school may be detrimental. Finally, parents must work with healthcare providers and school personnel to identify stressors, depression symptoms, and peer concerns that may be negatively affecting their child.

What Should I Tell the School Nurse?

The school nurse plays an important role in the care of a child with headaches. He or she usually keeps the medications for the child, encourages her to maximize non-drug treatment options, and communicates with her teachers, parents, and healthcare providers. The nurse should also keep track of headache-related absences and time lost during the school day for headaches. Above all, the nurse can act as an important advocate for your child.

When your child is diagnosed with migraine, set up a meeting with the school nurse to discuss your child's treatment plan. Be sure to discuss:

▶ *What medications your child should take when she has a headache.* Be sure to provide a supply of both over-the-counter and prescription medications she may be using. It is best to have a step-by-step treatment strategy available for the nurse.

▶ *What non-drug treatments you want the nurse to encourage during a visit.* This might include using an ice pack or heating pad on the neck, dimming the lights, relaxation techniques, and stretching exercises. If your child practices relaxation techniques or biofeedback using an audio recording, provide a copy to be kept in the nurse's office.

▶ *How long you expect your child to stay at the nurse's office.* Remind the nurse that migraines in children and adolescents are generally resolved within an hour or two, so there is generally no need to send the child home for the day. Reinforce that one of the primary goals is to keep the child in school.

▶ *Whether your child usually vomits* with a migraine, so that access to a toilet or emesis basin can be routine. Nausea is quite common in children with migraines. If nausea medications are part of the treatment plan, they should be made available to the school to provide to your child. Most migraine sufferers feel much better after vomiting and should not need to be sent home because they

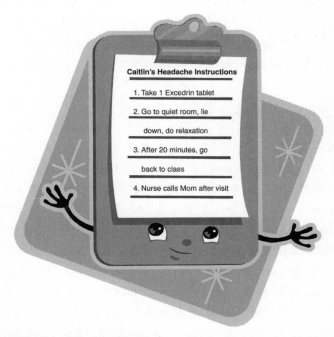

Give specific, detailed, written instructions for your child with migraines to the school nurse.

threw up. If the child has medication to treat nausea, encourage the school nurse to give it to her ASAP after nausea develops.

▶ *How you would like to be contacted about nurse visits.* Learning when and how often your child is visiting the nurse for headaches, even when she successfully returns to class after brief visits, can provide valuable information about migraine frequency and what might be triggering your child's migraines. Many schools now routinely will notify the parents either by phone or email if their child is seen in the health room.

Sleep can be a potent headache reliever in children. Try having your child lie down for a 15- to 20-minute nap with her next migraine. If she wakes headache-free or with a substantially relieved headache, let the school nurse know that a short nap in the nurse's office may be helpful when your child has a headache. Be sure to reinforce that the nurse should wake the child after 20 minutes rather than permitting long naps. If your child feels the need for long naps during the day, make sure she is getting enough sleep each night by following the sleep recommendations at the end of this chapter.

What Should I Tell My Child's Teacher?

The child's teacher plays a key role as well. If the teacher understands that the child has migraines, and that a treatment plan has been agreed upon with the school nurse, the teacher is more likely to accept the migraine diagnosis and permit nurse visits when they are first requested, rather than delaying and risking the child becoming ill in front of classmates. Your child's teacher may also begin to recognize early symptoms that a headache episode may be developing (even before the child recognizes them), such as changes in skin coloration, yawning, or irritability, and encourage the child to do neck stretches or deep-breathing exercises to prevent escalation. The teacher can also help the child keep up with her work and, if necessary, provide flexible options to make up missed work. Finally, the teacher can be a good observer for psychosocial stressors, childhood depression symptoms, and peer issues.

In some circumstances, it may also be helpful to involve the school psychologist or guidance counselor to help identify school-related problems that may make successful treatment more difficult, such as peer pressure, bullying, child abuse, learning disabilities, alcohol and drug abuse, self-esteem issues, friend issues, and depression/anxiety. The psychologist may be able to help the child develop important coping strategies, as well as reinforce stress management skills.

MEDICATIONS FOR MIGRAINE

What Drugs Should Be Considered During Childhood and Adolescence?

Unlike adult headaches, the number of drugs that have been specifically tested for treating headaches in children is more limited.

Research studies on migraine—as for most conditions—typically exclude children and adolescents for two reasons. First, doctors generally like to see that a medication has a long track record of safety in adults before using it on a child. Second, research studies usually divide patients into a group that's treated with the drug being tested and a group that's being treated with a sugar pill or placebo. After the drug is tested, researchers look to see if people did better when they were taking the actual drug compared with the placebo. In general, about one in every three adults will get migraine relief from a placebo. Children and adolescents are much stronger placebo responders, so about half of youngsters will get migraine relief from a placebo. Because children can respond well to a placebo during research studies, it's much harder to show that the actual drug is better than a placebo. This may be related to the much shorter duration of headaches typically seen in children.

As a parent, you can take advantage of the added placebo benefit your child will likely get from any treatment by enhancing what is referred to as the *placebo effect*. The placebo effect is strongest when the patient believes the treatment is likely to be helpful. So, when you're talking to your child about headache treatments, say things like, "Your doctor prescribed a strong migraine medication for you to take when you get a bad migraine at school. This should help get rid of most of your headache, so you can go back to class after taking it." Avoid making negative or pessimistic comments like, "Well, you can try this, but it has never helped one of my headaches," or "I don't know if this will work, but I guess we can give it a try." Adding the benefits from any placebo response to the proven benefits from the actual drug will only enhance your child's pain relief.

Dosing medications for children and adolescents should always be discussed with your healthcare provider. Dosing both over-the-counter and prescription medications should be discussed with your healthcare provider when developing a treatment plan.

Treating Headache Episodes

A number of medications have been tested and proven effective for treating migraines in children and adolescents. Analgesics and triptans are effective for treating individual headache episodes, although dose adjustments may be needed depending on the child's age and weight. Individual agents that have been effectively used in young people include ibuprofen (Advil®, Motrin®), almotriptan (Axert®), rizatriptan (Maxalt®), sumatriptan (Imitrex®), and zolmitriptan (Zomig®).

Both ibuprofen and several fast-acting triptan drugs have been tested and found to be relatively safe and effective in children and adolescents.

Generally, triptans are administered to children and young adolescents at approximately half the starting adult dose. Teenagers who are close to adult size may need to follow adult dosing recommendations. Orally disintegrating triptans may be particularly useful in children as they don't require fluids to help with swallowing.

Many of the anti-nausea agents used in adults are also useful for children. Metoclopramide (Reglan®), prochlorperazine (Compazine®), and ondansetron (Zofran®) are the most commonly used medications for nausea. They are generally very well tolerated. Since nausea is often a prominent component of migraine episodes in children, finding an effective anti-nausea agent is usually very important to the success of the headache treatment program. Again, orally dissolving ondansetron may be an especially attractive option because water is not required to take this medication.

Rescue medications should be available for those infrequent occasions when other therapies haven't helped. Common anti-migraine rescue agents that can be used in children and adolescents include the antihistamines diphenhydramine (Benadryl®) and hydroxyzine (Vistaril®, Atarax®). Opioid or narcotic analgesics are rarely helpful for migraine and should generally be avoided in children and adolescents.

Preventive Therapy

Just as in adults, taking analgesics or other medications designed to treat individual headache episodes more than 2 days per week can lead to the development of medication overuse or rebound headaches. For this reason, children and adolescents with frequent headaches may need prevention therapy.

Studies evaluating prevention drugs in children are limited. Drugs that effectively prevent migraine that have been directly tested in young people include propranolol (Inderal®); the antidepressants amitriptyline (Elavil®) and trazodone (Desyrel®, Beneficat®); and the anti-seizure drugs valproate (Depakene®, Depacon®) and topiramate (Topamax®).

A study that compared migraine prevention in 120 children ages 3–15 years treated with either propranolol or valproate found that headache frequency was reduced by at least half in seven of ten children treated with either valproate or propranolol. A small study comparing headache improvement in 48 children with migraine treated with either valproate or topiramate likewise found that both treatments provided similar results. The anti-seizure drug levetiracetam (Keppra XR®) was effective in preventing migraines in two studies testing small numbers of youngsters (19 youth in one study and 20 in another); however, both valproate and topiramate have been more extensively studied in younger patients than has levetiracetam.

The prevention drugs propranolol and some drugs originally designed to treat mood disorders or epilepsy have been tested and found to be relatively safe and effective in children and adolescents.

Migraine prevention medications can be sedating. Children taking these medications should be monitored for problems with alertness, concentration, and school performance. The newer class of antidepressants called *selective serotonin reuptake inhibitors* (SSRIs) are sometimes used to treat migraines in adults, although they tend to be only modestly effective. Because SSRIs have been linked to a small but significantly increased risk of suicide in pediatric patients being treated for mood disorders, careful monitoring is required in young people using SSRI antidepressants.

NON-DRUG TREATMENTS FOR MIGRAINE

Can Kids Learn to Use Non-Drug Treatments?

Children are excellent candidates for non-drug treatment options. Perhaps because they are students, many young people readily learn and master non-drug techniques, generally getting even better headache relief than when these techniques are used by adults. For that reason, non-drug options should be encouraged for all children with headaches.

A variety of non-drug treatments have been directly tested in youngsters. Effective non-drug headache therapies for children and adolescents include relaxation, stress management, and biofeedback. Healthy lifestyle habits should also be encouraged, although research studies have not directly tested the benefits of these treatments in young people with headaches. Important lifestyle habits include:

▶ Daily aerobic exercise
▶ Eating regular, balanced meals and not skipping meals
▶ Maintaining good hydration, especially during sporting events
▶ Keeping a regular sleeping schedule

Identify Stress Factors in Your Child's Life

Many circumstances increase stress for children and adolescents. These may include:

▶ School coursework
▶ Difficulty interacting with a peer group
▶ Bullying
▶ Excessive after-school commitments
▶ Depression
▶ Anxiety
▶ Fears of health conditions or illness
▶ Family strife
▶ Sexual issues
▶ Drug exposure or pressure

Talk to your child about her individual concerns, and consider including your child's doctor, psychologist, or counselor in determining strategies for addressing significant problems. Many children with headaches benefit greatly from seeing a behavioral psychologist to learn relaxation and stress management techniques.

Sleep Recommendations

For good health, children and teens need to sleep more than the average adult. Unfortunately, most youngsters with headache have impaired sleep. In a study of over 1,000 students, poor sleep was identified as a headache trigger for one in three of those with headaches. By setting strict times for going to bed and getting up each day, you can help reduce the chances that sleep deficits are triggering your child's headaches.

How much sleep do young people need? Research indicates that:

▶ Elementary and middle school students need 10 hours each night.
▶ Teenagers need more than 9 hours of sleep each night.

TIPS TO MINIMIZE HEADACHES IN YOUNGSTERS

1. *Educate yourself and your child about migraine.* Let her know that migraines are a biological condition and that a lot of effective treatments are available.

2. *Make regular sleep a priority.* Kids need to sleep 9–10 hours each night.

3. *Avoid over-scheduling your child with too many extracurricular activities.* If she's spending more than 2 hours each day in extracurricular activities, she should probably cut back on her commitments.

4. *Make meal time a priority.* Don't allow your child to skip meals.

5. *Make sure your child is well hydrated*, especially when involved in sports.

6. *Encourage her to practice and learn helpful pain management techniques*, such as relaxation, biofeedback, and stress management.

7. *Talk to your child about stress.* Overscheduling, pressures to succeed, bullying, peer relationships, and availability of alcohol and drugs are common stresses faced by many youngsters that can negatively impact headaches.

8. *Encourage daily aerobic exercise.* The World Health Organization recommends 60 minutes of moderate to vigorous physical activity daily for children 5–17 years old. Exercise is a great way to help reduce pain, because it results in a release of endorphins, your body's natural pain killers. Exercise also helps reduce stress, build confidence and self-esteem, and provide an avenue for positive socialization with peers.

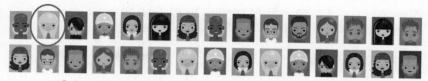

**Only one in every twenty-five young people gets the necessary
9 hours of sleep each night.**

How many adolescents get enough sleep?

One study of adolescents with headache showed that only one of every 25 youths got at least 9 hours of sleep on school nights, with an average sleep time of 7½ hours.

Set Up a Strict Sleep Program for Your Child

▶ Establish regular times for going to bed with lights off and getting up in the morning. Make sure this totals at least 9 hours.

▶ Don't let your child watch television or play computer games after bedtime. Researchers at the German Sport University in Cologne, Germany, showed that excessive television viewing or computer game-playing resulted in sleep impairments. Make time to prepare for sleep. It is difficult for the brain to shut off quickly—some wind-down time is usually necessary.

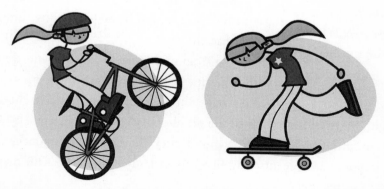

Youngsters should exercise at least 1 hour every day.

NUTRITIONAL SUPPLEMENTS FOR MIGRAINE

Which Natural Products Have Been Shown to Help Kids?

Few vitamins, minerals, and herbs have been tested in children and teenagers. Always talk to your doctor before giving vitamin supplements, minerals, or herbs to your child or adolescent.

Nutritional supplements that have been specifically tested and shown to be effective for reducing migraine in youngsters include: butterbur (or *Petasites hydrides*), coenzyme Q10 (CoQ10), magnesium, and riboflavin.

In one study of butterbur testing young people with migraine, taking 25–75 mg (depending on the child's weight) of butterbur extract twice daily for 4 months decreased the number of migraines by 63 percent. Both children and teenagers experienced a similar degree of migraine relief with butterbur. As in adults, the most common side effect was burping. This medication can be ordered online at www.migraineaide.com.

Researchers tested 1,550 pediatric patients at a headache specialty clinic for CoQ10 deficiency. They found that one in three had low levels, and these children were given CoQ10 supplemental at doses of 1–3 mg per kilogram of body weight per day (or about .5 to 1.4 mg per pound of body weight). Headache frequency was reduced by 50 percent in almost half of the children.

Nutritional remedies that have been proven to reduce headaches in young people include butterbur, coenzyme Q10, magnesium, and riboflavin.

One large study treated children and teens with migraine with magnesium for 4 months, with dosage varying according to each child's weight. Magnesium decreased the number of days with migraine by 45 percent, and also decreased their severity. Tension-type headache in children and adolescents may also be substantially reduced with magnesium supplements.

Riboflavin was given to a group of 41 youngsters with migraine in a research study, at a dose 200 or 400 mg of riboflavin daily for at least 3 months. Headache frequency dropped by at least half in two-thirds of the children. Side effects were minimal.

PUTTING IT ALL TOGETHER

1. Educate yourself and your child about headaches. The more you know, the more empowered you and your child will feel. Resources for childhood headache sufferers are listed in Chapter 9.

2. Have your child keep track of her headaches using a headache calendar or diary.

3. Work with the child's school nurse, teacher and, if necessary, the school counselor or psychologist. Everyone must be on the same page with goals and expectations for headache treatment.

4. Make regular follow-up appointments with your child's healthcare provider. If your healthcare provider doesn't hear from you, often she will assume that things are going well.

5. Maximize non-drug treatments. Make sure that the child doesn't skip meals, stays well-hydrated, and has regular, consistent sleeping and waking times. And avoid scheduling too many extracurricular activities.

6. Treat headache pain early and aggressively. Have medications available at all times.

7. Treat nausea early and aggressively.

8. Make staying in school a priority. Missing school can lead to the development of school avoidance and other problems.

9. Monitor your child's medication use. Be aware of the possibility that medication overuse or rebound headaches may develop if your child regularly uses medications to treat individual headache episodes more than 2 days per week.

10. If headaches are frequent, discuss adding preventive therapy with your child's doctor.

Summary

▶ Chronic headaches are common in children and adolescents and can result in substantial days lost from attending school.

▶ Young people are most likely to have headaches during school hours.

▶ Maintaining school attendance is a top goal for headache treatment in young people.

▶ Headache diagnosis and management strategies should be discussed with the child, the child's teacher, and the school nurse to help make treatments consistent at home and at school.

▶ Headaches can be effectively treated in children and adolescents with non-drug pain management skills such as relaxation, biofeedback, and stress management; exercise; healthy scheduling such as a regular sleep pattern, eating three meals a day, and avoiding excessive extracurricular commitments; medications; and some nutritional supplements.

5

Controlling Menstrual Migraine

One of the most significant hormonal milestones in a woman's life is the onset of menses. Adolescent girls usually begin the cycle of ovulation, falling estrogen, and menstrual bleeding at around age 11–12. This cycle will continue through most of their adulthood, interrupted only by pregnancy.

Estrogen and other hormones increase and then begin to cycle at puberty, resulting in a surge in headache activity for many girls. The cycling of hormones and other body chemicals with monthly menstrual periods often causes a marked increase in headache frequency and severity with menstrual flow and, to a lesser extent, mid-cycle with ovulation. A variety of factors contribute to a reduced headache threshold with menstruation:

- ▶ Falling hormone levels
- ▶ Low magnesium
- ▶ Increases in substances called prostaglandins that make pain receptors more sensitive
- ▶ Changes in muscle tension
- ▶ Increased susceptibility to headache triggers

If you or your daughter experience an increase in headache or clustering of your headaches around your menstrual periods, you or she

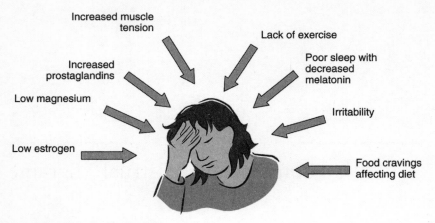

Factors contributing to menstrual migraine.

might benefit from tailoring your treatment to include therapies specifically designed to target menstrual migraine.

WHAT IS MENSTRUAL MIGRAINE?

Headaches are associated with menses for about three of every five women with migraines. Menstrual migraine is generally considered to be triggered by a drop in estrogen levels that begins about 2 days before the beginning of the menstrual period. Headaches that are triggered by this change in estrogen are most likely to occur during the 5 days around the beginning of each menstrual period—starting 2 days before menstrual bleeding begins and through the first 3 days of menstrual flow. This time around the beginning of your menstrual period is called the *perimenstrual* time. (The prefix *peri* means *around*.)

The perimenstrual time *includes the few days before your period begins and the first few days of menstrual bleeding.*

You might have headaches on each of these days or on only a few of them. Women whose migraines occur *only* during these 5 days for at least two of every three cycles are defined as having *pure menstrual migraine*. Only about 15 percent of women have migraines that occur exclusively during these 5 days.

Most women have headaches that occur with their menstrual cycles *and* on non-menstrual days. If your migraines typically worsen around your menstrual period, but also occur when you're not having your period, you can be diagnosed with *menstrually related migraine*. About half of women with migraine have this type of migraine activity. In general, migraine attacks without an aura tend to occur more frequently during the time around the menstrual period.

Menstrually Related Migraine

If I have migraines with my period and also at other times, why should I focus on my menstrual migraines?

Migraine attacks aggravated by your menstrual period are typically more severe than attacks that happen at other times of the month. Compared with migraine headaches that occur at other times of the month, menstrual migraines tend to be more frequent, more disabling, and less responsive to medications.

Menstrual migraines can be diagnosed when you have a marked increase in headache frequency or severity that occurs when estrogen levels drop—from 2 days before the onset of menstrual bleeding through the first 3 days of your period.

Many women find that those treatments that work well to control their usual non-menstrual headaches are less effective for menstrual attacks. For this reason, you often need special treatment for your menstrual migraines.

The *good* news about menstrual migraines is that they are generally predictable. Because you can often identify when these migraines are likely to occur, you can use medication and non-drug treatments to try to effectively prevent or minimize their severity.

Diagnosing Menstrual Migraine

How can I be sure if I'm having menstrual migraines?

In order to determine if your headaches are related to your menstrual periods, you will need to keep a headache diary for 2 to 3 months.

Be sure to record both headache activity and when your menstrual periods occur. You may notice one of these patterns:

▶ Your headaches occur *only* around your menstrual periods: You have pure menstrual migraine.

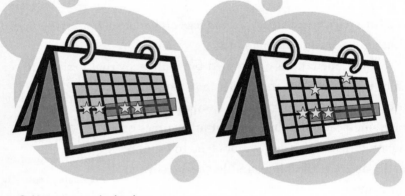

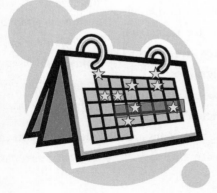

Monitor your migraines and menstrual periods with diaries. Migraines are marked by stars and menstrual days by the long shaded box.

▶ Your headaches become more frequent and more severe around your menstrual periods, but you also have headaches at other times of the month: You have menstrually related migraine.

▶ Your headaches don't seem to be any worse around your menstrual period. They seem to be scattered randomly throughout the month, sometimes occurring with your menstrual periods but just as likely to occur on non-menstrual days: You don't have menstrual migraines.

▶ Your headaches typically occur or get much worse during the placebo week of your birth control pills: Your migraines are likely to be aggravated by the estrogen drop that occurs during the placebo week. Talk to your doctor about modifying your contraceptive therapy.

Menses is a potent migraine trigger. Help decrease your migraine threshold during your period by reducing your exposure to other possible common triggers— practice stress management, relaxation, and exercise; maintain a regular sleep pattern; stay hydrated; and don't skip meals.

NON-DRUG OPTIONS FOR MENSTRUAL MIGRAINE

How can I use non-drug treatments for menstrual migraines?

Several non-drug treatments have been specifically tested for the treatment of menstrual migraine. Relaxation therapy, including biofeedback, has been shown to help reduce menstrual migraines. Similar to non-menstrual migraine, acupuncture is not effective for menstrual migraine.

Healthy lifestyle practices may be particularly important during the perimenstrual time. Headache triggers can be additive—two or more triggers can combine to lower the threshold more than either one alone. Around the time of your menstrual period, changes in hormones, magnesium levels, and prostaglandins, for example, can act as important headache triggers. Because the physiology of menstruation causes a number of triggers you can't control, it's especially important that you minimize those triggers that you *can* control. During the few days before you expect your period and for the first few days of menstrual bleeding, make an extra effort to not skip meals, avoid possible dietary triggers such as red wine, and get an adequate amount of sleep, with regular bed and waking times. Even if you feel bloated with your period, don't skip meals or limit the amount of water you drink—fasting and dehydration are important migraine triggers. If you don't regularly exercise and practice relaxation techniques, your perimenstrual days can be an important time to add daily relaxation, stretching exercises, and aerobic exercise to your routine.

MEDICATION OPTIONS FOR MENSTRUAL MIGRAINE

Which drugs work and when should I take them in my cycle?

You can still use your regular migraine therapies if you have menstrual migraines. If your usual treatments aren't helpful for your menstrual attacks, you may want to include therapy that is specifically directed to those high-susceptibility headache days around each menstrual period. In many cases, you can prevent menstrual migraines from occurring by adding a brief course of a prevention therapy.

You will generally need to take prevention medications for several weeks or months before you will notice an improvement in non-menstrual migraines. Interestingly, however, a short course of a new prevention therapy or a temporary dosage increase in your usual daily prevention therapy around the time of your menstrual periods often successfully reduces menstrually triggered migraines.

Effective therapy to prevent migraine aggravation with your menstrual period is call *mini-prophylaxis*. *Prophylaxis* is another word for prevention, so mini-prophylaxis means a short course of a prevention therapy. Menstrual migraines may improve by using mini-prophylaxis

MINI-PROPHYLAXIS OF MENSTRUAL HEADACHE

Consider mini-prophylaxis only if your headache diary consistently shows a strong link between migraine aggravation and your menstrual periods.

▶ *Mini-prophylaxis with perimenstrual hormone therapy:* 1.5 mg transdermal estrogen patch worn for 7 days, starting 2–5 days before your period is expected to begin

▶ *Mini-prophylaxis with standard headache therapies:* All medications should be used at standard migraine treatment doses (unless otherwise specified by your healthcare provider) for 2–3 days before the expected menstrual period and during the first 2–4 days of menses. Standard acute headache medications include:

- Nonsteroidal anti-inflammatory drugs (for example, naproxen sodium 550 mg twice daily with food or mefenamic acid (Ponstel®) 500 mg three times daily with food)

- 1 mg naratriptan (Amerge®) twice daily

- 2.5 mg frovatriptan (Frova®) once or twice daily

- Sumatriptan (Imitrex®) 25 mg three times daily

▶ Standard headache preventive medications include:

- Beta-blockers, such as propranolol (Inderal®)

- Antidepressants, such as amitriptyline (Elavil®) or imipramine (Tofranil®)

- Calcium-channel blockers, such as verapamil (Calan® and Isoptin®), and flunarizine (Sibelium®; not available in the United States)

- Neurostabilizing antiepileptics, such as topiramate (Topamax®)

If you're already taking a prevention therapy, you may increase your daily dose of that prevention for the week before your expected menstrual period. Be sure to talk to your doctor before adjusting doses of any of your prescription medications.

with hormonal therapy or standard migraine drugs. Remember—the same restrictions for using medications and side effects that were discussed in Chapter 3 will also apply to using these same medications when treating menstrual migraine. Also, if you increase your medication dose during the perimenstrual period, you may experience more side effects with this dose increase. Always talk to your healthcare provider before starting any new medication regimen.

If you are already taking a migraine prevention medication, talk to your doctor about temporarily increasing the dose during the perimenstrual time. For example, if you regularly take topiramate 25 mg at bedtime every day as a migraine prevention therapy, you might try increasing this dose to 50 mg at bedtime up to 5 days before you expect your period to start and for the first 2 days of menstrual bleeding. Then reduce your dose back to 25 mg for the remainder of the month. Again, be sure to consult with your healthcare provider before making any change in your usual medication regimen.

Some studies have evaluated the benefit of anti-estrogen therapy, such as danazol (Danocrine®) and tamoxifen (Soltamox®); the endometriosis treatment gonadotropin-releasing hormone agonist followed by estrogen add-back therapy; and the dopamine mimic bromocriptine (Parlodel®, Cycloset®). These treatments may have serious side effects and should be considered as experimental therapies. They should probably only be considered after consultation with your gynecologist.

Hormonal Approaches to Menstrual Migraine

Blunting the significant drop in estrogen just before menses sometimes can help reduce menstrual migraine. An estrogen patch, pill, or gel can effectively decrease the steep decline in estrogen and minimize headache symptoms. In general, transdermal estrogen in a patch or gel form is the most effective for menstrual migraine, because it provides the steadiest concentration of estrogen. Estrogen should generally be started up to 5 days before you expect your period in order to effectively blunt the usual drop in estrogen.

Some women use estrogen-containing oral contraceptive pills (birth control pills) to help reduce menstrual symptoms, including menstrual migraine. Traditional oral contraceptives include 3 weeks of active pills containing hormones and a 4th week of placebo or sugar pills that don't. (The reason for taking the placebo pills is to keep you in the habit of taking your birth control pill every day.) Estrogen levels drop during the placebo week, and you will have menstrual bleeding that is just like a normal period. In some cases, your doctor may suggest that you skip the placebo week of your birth control pills—starting the next pill pack after you finish the 3 active pill weeks. You may take only active pills for 2 or 3 months before returning to using the placebo week and having a period. Taking a *monophasic* pill (those with the same dose of estrogen in all tablets) in the lowest possible estrogen dose—typically 20 mcg—continuously without placebo pills is often the best way to prevent menstrual headaches with hormonal therapy.

Many people wonder if taking estrogen continuously for several months without a break is harmful. Traditional birth control packs have a placebo week to allow for estrogen withdrawal that leads to shedding of the endometrial lining, resulting in menstrual bleeding. It was thought in the past that a woman had to shed her uterine lining every month to reduce the risk of endometrial or uterine cancer. This has been shown in recent years not to be necessary. Often when a woman takes a low-dose estrogen-containing birth control pill continuously, she will notice spotting. If this continues or is heavy, her healthcare provider may recommend that she stop the estrogen-containing pill temporarily for 5–7 days to induce a period. Alternatively, the provider may try to induce a period by having her take progesterone for 3–5 days. In either case, the estrogen-containing birth control pills can be restarted when the bleeding significantly slows or stops.

Certain women should *avoid* estrogen-containing birth control pills because of increased risk of serious side effects:

► Smokers—because of a higher risk of stroke

► Individuals who have migraine with aura—because of a higher risk of stroke

► Those with a personal or family history of blood clots—estrogen also increases the risk of clotting

► Women with breast cancer or a family history of breast cancer— estrogen can increase the risk of developing breast cancer. Interestingly, taking birth control pills that include both estrogen and a progestin has been shown to reduce your risk for developing ovarian cancer.

Progesterone-only birth control pills (sometimes referred to as the *mini pill*), progesterone-only injection (Depo-Provera®), and an intrauterine device (IUD) that releases the synthetic progestogen hormone levonorgestrel (Mirena®) are less effective than combination pills at preventing ovulation, and may work as contraceptives by altering cervical mucous thickness. In general, progesterone-only preparations are less likely to influence menstrual migraine compared with estrogen-containing pills.

Oral Contraceptives and Migraine

What do I do if my birth control pills worsen my headache?

When headaches are aggravated by taking birth control pills, women usually notice that their worst headaches occur during the first few days of the placebo pills in the birth control pill pack. When you switch to the placebo pills, your estrogen level will drop. This is the same time of the month when you would normally have a drop in your estrogen level. By taking extra estrogen during the active pill weeks, the drop from the highest estrogen level your body experiences to the lowest level is more than before you started taking the pill. In general, the bigger the drop in estrogen, the more likely you are to have an aggravation of your migraines.

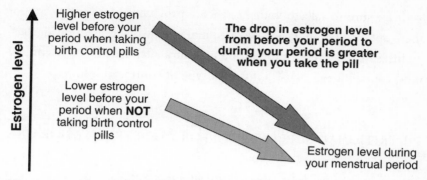

Higher estrogen level before your period when taking birth control pills

The drop in estrogen level from before your period to during your period is greater when you take the pill

Lower estrogen level before your period when **NOT** taking birth control pills

Estrogen level during your menstrual period

Estrogen level

Migraines are often triggered when estrogen levels fall from high to low levels.

Headache aggravation with birth control pills has been reported in up to half of all the women with migraine who have tried using them. In most cases, these women's headaches improve after stopping birth control pills; however, some women find that it takes up to a year after stopping before their headaches go back to the way they were before using this form of birth control. If your headaches have worsened with the use of birth control pills, you might discuss these strategies with your doctor:

▶ *Reduce the estrogen dose of the active pills.* If the everyday estrogen dose is lower, your body experiences less of a change from the highest level of estrogen that occurs during the weeks when you're taking active pills to the lowest estrogen level during the placebo week.

▶ *Supplement with additional low-dose estrogen during the placebo week.* Studies show benefit from adding 0.9 mg estrogen on each day of the placebo week.

▶ *Reduce the duration of the placebo week, including eliminating the placebo week from most cycles.* You might discard the placebo week pills from your oral contraceptives for 2 or 3 consecutive months and start your next pack with active pills when you would normally have been using the placebo pills from the previous pack. This will result in missing one or two periods before cycling back to the placebo week and having a regular cycle.

Be sure to talk to your healthcare provider before trying any of these options. If you have developed a marked worsening of headaches, an increase in aura symptoms, or a new aura after starting birth control pills, you will need to use a different type of contraception.

NUTRITIONAL SUPPLEMENTS FOR MENSTRUAL MIGRAINE

Do any natural products treat menstrual migraine?

Phytoestrogens are naturally occurring estrogens, and they are sometimes called "dietary" estrogens. They have been shown to significantly reduce menstrual migraines, similar to using prescription estrogen supplementation.

Phytoestrogen supplements are chemically similar to the estrogens your body produces. Effective phytoestrogen treatment strategies that have been tested and shown to be effective in research studies include:

- ▶ Mini-prophylaxis with genistein 56 mg, plus daidzein 20 mg, 7 days before the expected menstrual period and 3 days of menses
- ▶ Soy extract 75 mg, dong quai extract 50 mg, plus black cohosh 25 mg twice daily

Magnesium taken 360 mg per day starting 2 weeks before menses and continued until your period begins has been used to treat the magnesium deficiency that occurs in many women with menstrual migraine. In one study, this approach resulted in a drop in the frequency of menstrual migraines by nearly half of those receiving this supplement.

Effective natural remedies for menstrual migraine include phytoestrogens, magnesium, and possibly melatonin.

Vitamins and herbs have not been tested specifically for menstrual migraine. Melatonin levels were shown to decrease during menses in women with menstrual migraine, suggesting that perimenstrual melatonin supplementation might be beneficial.

PUTTING IT ALL TOGETHER

A number of effective treatment strategies are available for patients with menstrual migraine, including:

1. Keep track of your headaches using a calendar or diary. Mark down when you have a headache, how severe the symptoms are, whether your usual treatment worked or not, and if you had your menstrual period that day. Keeping track of your headaches through two or three menstrual cycles will help you identify whether you have menstrual migraines.

2. Maximize your use of non-drug migraine prevention strategies during your perimenstrual time.

Talk with your healthcare provider about various treatment strategies if you find that your headaches are consistently associated with having your period. You might consider perimenstrual treatments with hormones, standard migraine treatments, or natural remedies such as phytoestrogens, magnesium, and possibly melatonin.

SUMMARY

- Record your headache and menstrual patterns in a diary for 2–3 months to help determine if you have menstrual migraines.
- Menstrual migraines are often more severe, more frequent, and more difficult to treat than migraines occurring at other times of the month.
- If you have menstrual migraines, and your periods are regular and predictable, you can try increasing your use of non-drug treatments or use medication mini-prophylaxis during your perimenstrual time to help reduce menstrual migraines.
- Perimenstrual treatment with estrogen supplements or standard migraine drugs has been shown in research studies to significantly reduce menstrual migraines.

6

Safe Treatment of Migraines During Pregnancy and Nursing

Becoming pregnant is one of the most exciting times in a woman's life, signaling her entry into motherhood. For patients with migraine, however, pregnancy can become a time of significant anxiety and apprehension. Pregnant women with migraine are likely to have many questions: *Will I have more headaches? Will I have to suffer? Can I take medication for the headaches? Will my migraine headaches harm the baby? Should I breastfeed? What can I do if I have a headache while breast-feeding?*

Fortunately, decades of research on headaches and pregnancy provide good answers to these types of questions. A variety of safe and effective treatments can be used when you're pregnant or breastfeeding. Ideally, maximizing non-drug options is important to reduce medication exposure for the baby. Most women prefer not to use medications during pregnancy unless absolutely necessary. While many headache sufferers intend to avoid medications when they learn they're pregnant, many will need to use migraine medications at some point before the baby is born. A recently published study of almost 3,500 women with migraine during the first 5 months of pregnancy found that three out of every four women used migraine medications during pregnancy. A little over half used analgesic pain medications, and one in four used a triptan.

Be sure to include headache management in your pregnancy planning discussions with your healthcare provider. It is best to discuss this before becoming pregnant, or during the very early stages of your pregnancy, when headaches are most likely to be worse. Even though migraines often improve as pregnancy progresses, it's important to develop a treatment plan in case they occur later in the pregnancy. It is also important to discuss the postpartum period well ahead of time, because an increase in headaches often occurs after delivery. Also, even though migraines are less likely to return when a woman breastfeeds, it is important to have a migraine plan established before delivery, so that nursing is not interrupted or unnecessarily abandoned.

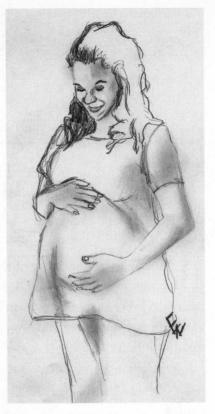

Make plans for likely migraine changes during pregnancy to reduce stress and anxiety about safely controlling your headaches.

Pre-Pregnancy Planning

Will I have to suffer?

As noted earlier, the best time to begin thinking about headache treatment during pregnancy is before you become pregnant. It is extremely important for women with migraines to avoid unplanned pregnancies. When you are ready for pregnancy, it is preferable that you be off all potentially unsafe medications. Also, it is best if your headache pattern is well controlled before you stop taking medications. When you are no longer using effective contraception—which can lead to pregnancy—you should use only medications that pose no significant harm to the developing fetus. In other words, you should be treated as if you are already pregnant.

Ideally, you and your physician should meet when pregnancy is first being considered to discuss general treatment principles during pregnancy. Many questions may come up in the pre-pregnancy planning stage. Many effective treatment options are available to pregnant women to treat symptoms such as pain and nausea. However, certain medications must be avoided because of their potential risk to the fetus. It is important to limit exposure to medications and maximize non-drug approaches, especially during the first trimester when the fetus is the most sensitive to medication.

Key Questions for Your Doctor

▶ *What should I ask about headache planning for pregnancy?* When you decide you're ready to start or add to your family, make an appointment for pre-pregnancy planning with your healthcare provider. You'll want to ask about what to expect during pregnancy headache-wise and whether you need to change your current migraine treatment.

▶ *What should I expect to happen to my migraines when I'm pregnant?* The *good* news is that migraines improve for most women during pregnancy:

- Headaches improve for about four in every five women by the third trimester.
- Headaches often don't improve until the early second trimester.
- Even if your headaches improve, you may continue to still have some troublesome headaches that will need treatment.

- Safe and effective treatments are available for use when you are trying to get pregnant and after you have become pregnant.

▶ *Will I need to change my migraine treatment? Should I make those changes now or wait until after I become pregnant?* The harmful effects of most medications on the developing baby are greatest at the beginning of pregnancy—often before you even realize you are pregnant. Therefore, it's best to start taking the treatments that are known to be safer during pregnancy for several months before trying to conceive. This time allows your body a chance to rid itself of any potentially harmful medications before you become pregnant. It also gives you a chance to make sure the new treatment will control your headaches. Ideally, you will have been stable on a successful, safe headache regimen for several months before becoming pregnant.

▶ *Shouldn't I try to not use any headache medications when I'm pregnant?* Ideally, you will only need to use non-drug treatment throughout your time of conception and pregnancy. The reality, however, is that most women who have migraine during pregnancy will need to use some medication. A recent survey of almost 3,500 women during their first 5 months of pregnancy showed that three in four women used headache medication. Over half used an analgesic therapy, and one in four used a triptan. Understanding which medications offer the best combination of safety and effectiveness for you and your baby will help you make the best choices for you.

Babies born to women with migraine have no identified increased risk for congenital malformations, low birth weight, or premature birth.

▶ *Will my having migraines harm the baby?* Fortunately, most babies born to mothers with migraine are generally healthy, normal weight, and born on time—even if Mom has severe migraines during pregnancy. There is no apparent increased risk for developing congenital malformations (birth defects) when Mom has migraines. So relax and enjoy your pregnancy!

Controlling your headaches during pregnancy is important for you *and* your baby. If your migraines become severe, you may become very nauseated. Severe nausea can lead to dehydration and poor nutrition that can affect your baby. You will learn about safer treatments for migraines and nausea in this chapter to help you treat headaches when you're pregnant.

▶ *Will having migraines complicate my pregnancy?* Most women with migraine have normal pregnancies and give birth to healthy babies. Migraine sufferers are at slightly higher risk for some pregnancy-related health problems. They are somewhat more likely to develop pregnancy-related hypertension. If your blood pressure becomes too high during pregnancy, you may develop pre-eclampsia and eclampsia. Women with pre-eclampsia have high blood pressure, extra protein in their urine, and fluid retention. If blood pressure becomes too high during pregnancy, it can sometimes lead to eclampsia, which is associated with an increased risk of having seizures and is treated by delivering the baby. Pre-eclampsia affects about five in every 100 pregnancies, while full-blown eclampsia only occurs in about five of every 10,000 pregnancies. The risk is still quite low in women with migraine, but it is slightly higher. Migraine, especially migraine with aura, has also been linked to an increased risk for developing strokes during pregnancy. Luckily strokes are very rare during pregnancy, affecting about three in every 10,000 pregnancies. Again, this risk is only slightly higher in women with migraine.

> *Women with migraines are at slightly increased risk for developing pre-eclampsia, eclampsia, and strokes, although these events are quite uncommon.*

▶ *What can I do to avoid pregnancy complications?* The best way to reduce your risk of these rare pregnancy-related complications is to keep yourself as healthy as possible and maintain good prenatal care. Eat right, stay active, and avoid harmful habits such as cigarette smoking. These are much bigger risk factors for high blood pressure and stroke than your migraines! If you do have a slight increase in your blood pressure, don't panic—your doctor may prescribe changes in your diet and routine to help get your blood pressure back down. Be sure to follow this advice—it's important for you and your baby!

▶ *What should I do before I get pregnant?* As discussed earlier, medication choices need to change with pregnancy to make sure you minimize risks to your baby. Before you start trying to get pregnant, you should talk to your doctor about your headache treatment. You will need to:

- Learn about safe and effective non-drug treatments that you can use to control headaches throughout your pregnancy and after delivery.

STEPS TO TAKE BEFORE BECOMING PREGNANT

1. Stop smoking.

2. Stop drinking alcohol completely.

3. Keep track of headaches using a diary (see Chapter 3).

4. If your headaches have been controlled for at least 6 months, talk to your doctor about weaning off of any preventive medications you're using.

5. Learn about what to expect with your headaches during pregnancy (see Chapter 2).

6. Learn effective non-medication options for pain (see Chapter 3).

7. Talk to your doctor about developing a medication plan during pregnancy and breastfeeding.

   a. Include safe treatments for headache and nausea.

   b. Be sure to get advice about using over-the-counter drugs and herbal or nutritional therapies.

8. Start prenatal vitamins with 400 mg of folate when you're trying to get pregnant.

- Make sure the headache medications you are using are safe for you to take when trying to get pregnant and throughout pregnancy. This reduces risks to the baby if you become pregnant while taking the medications.
- Try to get your headache pattern under as good control as possible before you become pregnant.
- Talk to your doctor before using any non-prescription medications and supplements to make sure they are safe during pregnancy.
- Take a multivitamin with *at least* 400 micrograms of folate every day. This helps to prevent spinal cord defects.

Remember that there are many safe and effective non-drug and drug treatments for you to use throughout pregnancy. Making treatment changes before you become pregnant is the best way to provide the safest treatments for your developing baby *and* to make sure you have an effective treatment regimen in place to adequately control your headaches.

PREGNANCY

Keeping It Safe for Baby

Congratulations! Pregnancy is a very exciting time involving many changes in your body. Effectively treating your headaches will allow you to better enjoy your pregnancy.

General recommendations for pregnant patients who have headaches:

▶ Quit smoking if you didn't do so in the pre-pregnancy period.
▶ Eat regular meals and snacks; don't skip meals, especially breakfast.
▶ Get a good night's sleep every night.
▶ Learn effective relaxation techniques.
▶ Learn headache-relieving neck stretching exercises.
▶ Don't use over-the-counter, herbal, or supplement remedies without first discussing them with your healthcare provider.

▶ Use safe and effective therapies to treat and relieve nausea.

▶ Develop a plan for treating severe headaches with your doctor. Make sure you know which treatments to try first.

▶ Talk to your doctor about prevention therapy if you are having frequent severe headaches.

Even if your headaches aren't a problem during pregnancy, talk to your doctor about safe treatment options that can be used if you decide to breastfeed your baby. Most women experience a return of their previous headaches after delivery. Fortunately, breastfeeding often delays the return of headaches. More headache treatment options are available when you're breastfeeding than during pregnancy, although some medications should be avoided. Work with your healthcare provider to develop a safe, effective treatment plan.

Key Questions for Your Doctor

What do I need to know about managing headaches during pregnancy?

As soon as you know that you're pregnant, make an appointment to talk to your doctor about your headaches.

You will need to ask your doctor about:

▶ Safe and effective non-drug treatments to control your headaches

▶ Which medications you can safely take for pain and nausea

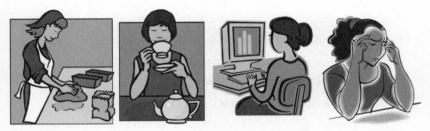

Migraine activity decreases by at least half during pregnancy in three out of four migraine sufferers who learn relaxation and biofeedback.

> ### Tips for Headache Treatment During Pregnancy
>
> ▶ Try to use effective non-drug options whenever possible.
>
> ▶ If you need medications, take safe treatments instead of suffering with a disabling headache.
>
> ▶ Most women with headaches will need to use headache medications at some point during their pregnancy.
>
> ▶ Develop a headache treatment plan with your doctor even if your migraines have improved with your pregnancy.
>
> ▶ Talk with your doctor before delivery about safe treatment options available during nursing.

▶ Which medications you can safely take to prevent headaches if this becomes necessary

▶ What to do if your headaches get worse

Let your doctor know:

▶ What your current headache pattern is like

▶ If there has been any recent change in your headaches

▶ If you are having any other medical problems besides headaches

▶ What over-the-counter medications you are taking

▶ What supplements, vitamins, minerals, and herbs you are taking

▶ What prescription medications you are taking and who prescribed them

It is important to realize that you are not expected to suffer with headaches during pregnancy. Headaches improve for four in every five women during pregnancy, so the odds are good that your headaches will get better. If not, many safe treatment options are available.

NON-DRUG THERAPIES

Will non-drug treatments really work when I'm pregnant?

Pregnancy is a great time to get motivated about incorporating effective non-drug migraine treatments (see Chapter 3).

Relaxation techniques, dietary regulation, and sleep regulation are especially important when you're pregnant. Other healthy lifestyle habits are also important, such as avoiding excess caffeine, stopping nicotine, and keeping physically active. Switch from high-impact to low-impact exercise, and talk to your doctor about starting any new exercise routine. Continue to practice stress management techniques— you'll be happy you've mastered them after the baby is born, when life may become even more hectic!

Relaxation Techniques

Relaxation and biofeedback have been found to be helpful during pregnancy and nursing. In a controlled research study, women who were having difficult headaches during pregnancy were treated with relaxation and biofeedback or a placebo treatment of just spending time with a therapist but not learning any pain management skills. Headache activity decreased by half or more in 73 percent of the women who learned relaxation and biofeedback, but only by 29 percent in those receiving the placebo treatment. This improvement continued throughout pregnancy and into the months after delivery. Almost 70 percent of women still reported headache improvement 1 year after their baby was born. These techniques really work!

Diet

Nutritional needs increase during pregnancy and when nursing. Make sure you maintain adequate nutrition by eating regular, well-balanced meals and snacks throughout the day. Fasting has consistently been linked to headache aggravation, so don't skip meals—especially when you're pregnant or nursing. Eating a restricted diet to reduce headaches is *not* recommended when you're pregnant or breastfeeding. Following a strict headache restrictive diet reduces migraines for only about one in three migraine sufferers. In addition, restrictive diets may unnecessarily limit nutritious foods, such as calcium-rich dairy foods and vitamin-rich fruits and vegetables. Instead, focus more on making sure you're eating regularly throughout the day and filling those meals with healthy foods.

Skipping meals is a potent headache trigger. Be sure to eat regularly.

Drink Plenty of Fluids

Dehydration is another important headache trigger. In general, people should drink 1–1.5 liters of water for every 1,000 calories eaten. If you're eating a 2,000-calorie diet, you need to drink 2–3 liters of water every day. Pregnant women generally need to increase their daily calorie intake by about 300 calories during the second trimester. This means that you'll need to drink an additional half liter of water each day.

Good hydration is important for your overall health and that of your developing baby. Good hydration is important to maintain healthy amniotic fluid around the growing baby. Furthermore, dehydration has been linked to an increased risk for pre-term labor.

Because dehydration can also be a potent headache trigger, staying hydrated may help to reduce your headaches. In a small study, non-pregnant adults with frequent headache were randomly assigned to one of two treatment groups. One group was instructed to add an extra half-liter of fluid to their normal beverage intake three times a day. The other group was given a sugar pill as a placebo control group. After 3 months, headache

Drink 8 to 10 glasses of water each day during pregnancy and breastfeeding. When you're nursing, drink one glass of water with each meal plus a glass of water every time you nurse your baby.

Headache Number   **Headache Severity**   **Headache Duration**

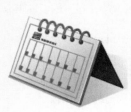

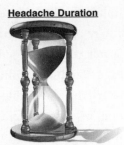

23 percent better with fluids   13 percent better with fluids   17 percent better with fluids
10 percent better with placebo   28 percent worse with placebo   no change with placebo

Effects of increasing fluid intake on headaches.

diaries were compared. Increasing daily fluid intake by 1.5 liters daily resulted in modest reductions in headache activity.

Take Prenatal Vitamins

It is important to take a daily prenatal vitamin with folate (also called *folic acid*). Research proves that women taking prenatal vitamins with folate have a lower risk of having babies with birth defects affecting the heart, arms and legs, or spinal cord (spina bifida). The Centers for Disease Control (CDC) and other public health organizations recommend that all women capable of becoming pregnant should get 400 micrograms of folic acid daily. This can be achieved by diets that include folate-enriched bread, cereal, rice, or pasta; lentils, legumes, leafy green vegetables, and citrus fruits; or with a vitamin supplement. To make certain you're getting enough folate, most doctors recommend taking a vitamin supplement with folate when you're pregnant or trying to get pregnant.

Getting 400 micrograms of folic acid daily reduces your baby's risk for birth defects.

Sleep

Poor sleep has been linked to an increased risk for headaches in general, and headache sufferers are encouraged to sleep 6–8 hours each night to

Out of 100 women, how many had *restless sleep?*

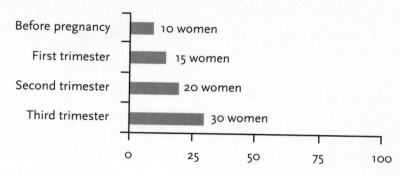

Out of 100 women, how many *slept soundly all night?*

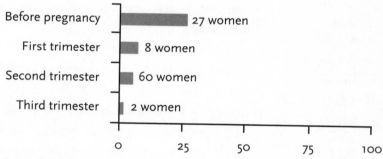

Sleep disturbances during pregnancy.

reduce headache risk. Regulating sleep may be particularly helpful during pregnancy, because pregnant women are more likely to report sleep disturbances. A study that followed 325 women throughout pregnancy evaluated sleep patterns before pregnancy and during each trimester. Although the total number of hours women slept didn't change during pregnancy, they were more likely to have restless sleep and wake up during the night as pregnancy progressed.

The sleep strategies described in Chapter 3 should be used to help improve sleep during pregnancy. Diphenhydramine (Benadryl®) is considered to be relatively safe, and you can talk to your doctor about using it occasionally during pregnancy. Be sure to read the drug labels, because diphenhydramine may be combined with analgesics such as acetaminophen (Tylenol®). Taking too much analgesic can result in medication overuse headaches, so use plain diphenhydramine if you don't need a painkiller. If you can't sleep for a prolonged period of time, such as four nights in a row, talk to your doctor.

Obstructive Sleep Apnea

Sleep apnea is an interruption in your breathing during sleep. *Obstructive* sleep apnea is the most common type of sleep apnea, caused by blockage of the upper airway. People with obstructive sleep apnea often report loud snoring. Your sleeping partner is likely to tell you that you snore loudly or stop breathing periodically during your sleep. Being overweight increases your risk for obstructive sleep apnea.

Talk to your doctor about sleep apnea if you snore loudly or someone tells you that you stop breathing periodically when you sleep.

Obstructive sleep apnea in a pregnant woman has been linked to distress in her developing baby. In a small study, 35 pregnant women who reported snoring or apnea were tested with sleep recordings and baby monitoring during sleep. Only four of the women were actually diagnosed with obstructive sleep apnea, suggesting only about one in every ten women with snoring or apnea will probably have this problem. Three of the four babies of mothers with obstructive sleep

---

FACTORS THAT SUGGEST OBSTRUCTIVE SLEEP APNEA

▶ Loud snoring (partner may have to sleep in another room)

▶ Witnessed apnea (stopped breathing)

▶ Excessive daytime fatigue

▶ High blood pressure (systolic blood pressure over 140 or diastolic blood pressure over 90)

▶ Large neck size (more than size 16 in a woman)

apnea showed signs of distress during Mom's apnea episodes, with slowing of the heart beat recording in the baby. In addition, babies born to women with obstructive sleep apnea had lower birth weights and Apgar scores (health scores shortly after birth). It's important that you talk to your doctor about an evaluation for obstructive sleep apnea if you have problems with snoring or have periods where you appear to stop breathing (sleep apnea).

Nausea

Nausea is most common during the first trimester and can be quite severe at times. Unfortunately, migraine is also most likely to be more frequent and severe during the first trimester, and migraine may increase nausea complaints. Dehydration can be a potent trigger for headaches. Nausea should be minimized to reduce disability, maximize good nutrition, and prevent dehydration.

Dietary modifications and acupressure point stimulation can help reduce mild to moderate nausea during pregnancy without medication.

Dietary adjustments can help reduce pregnancy-related nausea. Nauseated patients should avoid exposure to strong odors and drink bland liquids. Try diluting carbonated beverages and juices 1:1 with water. Nausea may also be curbed by snacking on easily digested, bland foods, such as crackers, applesauce, bananas, rice, and pasta.

Acupressure over the wrist can also relieve nausea. Find the P6 acupressure point, located in the middle of your arm between the tendons and

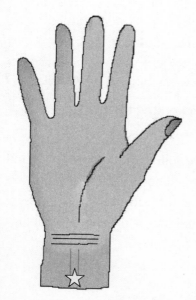

The star show the nausea-relief P6 acupressure point.

TIPS FOR TREATING NAUSEA DURING PREGNANCY

▶ Drink small amounts of cold, clear, and carbonated liquids between meals. Try to include ginger ale or lemon-lime soda, clear broth, juice diluted with water, gelatin, electrolyte drinks (such as Gatorade™ and Pedialyte™), and popsicles.

▶ When nausea has improved, move on to the BRAT diet: **B**ananas, **R**ice, **A**pplesauce, and **T**oast. Eat only small portions.

▶ Choose salty over sweet foods.

▶ Avoid hot, spicy, fried, greasy, or fatty food.

▶ If odors make you feel sick, use prepared or frozen foods, or let someone else do the cooking. You can also try using a nose clip to minimize breathing in troublesome odors.

▶ Eat in a cool, well-ventilated room away from where the food was prepared.

▶ Eat slowly.

▶ Iron supplements can increase nausea and may need to be temporarily reduced.

▶ An empty stomach may aggravate nausea, so eat frequent snacks, as soon as you feel hungry.

▶ Keep dry crackers by your bedside. Eat a few crackers in the morning before rising and then sit upright in bed for a few minutes before getting up to reduce the feeling of nausea that occurs with an empty stomach.

about two to three finger widths above your wrist crease. Deeply and firmly make circular motions over this area for several minutes. Over-the-counter Sea-Band™ wristbands can also activate this acupressure point and reduce nausea. These wristbands have a firm nodule that puts pressure over the P6 acupressure point for nausea.

HEADACHE MEDICATIONS

Which drugs are safe to use when you're pregnant?

You must consult with your doctor before using any drugs, supplements, or herbal preparations during pregnancy.

The Food and Drug Administration (FDA) helps to rate the safety of medications for all Americans. The most widely used tool for evaluating drug safety during pregnancy in the United States is the FDA's safety rating system. The system rates medication risk using categories A, B, C, D, and X, using information from studies in both animals and humans. Although these FDA pregnancy-risk categories have been a standard for many years, the agency is currently proposing to eliminate this rating system in favor of providing more detailed descriptions of pregnancy safety information for each drug.

Another system for rating drug safety during pregnancy is the Teratogen Information System (TERIS). A *teratogen* is a drug that causes birth defects. TERIS uses ratings of *no*, *minimal*, or *unlikely* risk for drugs that are likely to have received an FDA A or B rating; *undetermined* risk for FDA C drugs; and *small*, *moderate*, or *high* risk for FDA D or X drugs. Most healthcare providers generally agree that FDA categories A and B are relatively safe to take during pregnancy, and that D and X drugs should be limited or avoided. Unfortunately, about two in

---

TIPS FOR USING MIGRAINE DRUGS DURING PREGNANCY

► Don't medicate mild headaches.

► Treat nausea to avoid dehydration.

► Select safe drugs for treating migraines and nausea.

► Use the lowest effective dose.

► Use drugs for the shortest time possible.

► Especially minimize drug use during the earlier stages of pregnancy.

every three drugs has received an FDA risk category rating of C—often because they have not been tested during pregnancy. As a result, in most cases, your healthcare provider will advise you to minimize drug exposure—except for those drugs that are needed to treat serious health problems, including disabling migraine.

It is often difficult to say that a medication is *completely* safe. Recommendations are usually for *safer* rather than 100-percent safe medications. This is clearly a balancing act—weighing the risk of using a medication against the risk of treating severe symptoms such as pain, nausea, and dehydration.

Because of the uncertainty with many drugs, it's generally best to concentrate on non-drug therapies during pregnancy, and only use drugs to treat more disabling headaches that do not respond to non-drug treatments. In general, risks to the baby are greatest during the

---

FDA PREGNANCY RISK CLASSIFICATION SYSTEM

FDA Risk Category	Safety Rating
A	These drugs are considered **safe** to use during pregnancy, based on controlled research studies in women.
B	These drugs are considered **likely to be safe**, but controlled studies in women have not been done to confirm safety.
C	These drugs are considered **possibly to be unsafe**. Problems may have been identified in animal studies, but there are no studies in women. Drugs that haven't been tested in either pregnant animals or women will also be given a "C" rating.
D	These drugs are considered **probably to cause problems** for some exposed babies, but the drugs may still be used during pregnancy when the mother needs to treat a serious or life-threatening health problem and safer treatments won't work.
X	These drugs **will likely cause** problems for some exposed babies and **should be avoided** during pregnancy.

earlier stages of pregnancy, so early pregnancy is a particularly important time for limiting medication exposures.

Always let your delivery staff at the hospital know if you've been using any medications during pregnancy, so that the pediatrician can be prepared to support your baby, if needed.

Acute Treatments: Analgesics

Acetaminophen

Although acetaminophen is generally less effective for treating headache than aspirin or nonsteroidal anti-inflammatory drugs (NSAIDs, such as aspirin, ibuprofen [Motrin®], and naproxen [Naprosyn®, Aleve®]), it's safer during pregnancy. There is no increased risk of miscarriage with acetaminophen. Large population studies show no long-term effects in babies exposed to acetaminophen. It may be safely used throughout pregnancy.

Acetaminophen is very safe during pregnancy, and should be considered your first-line acute medication treatment. It is available in a variety of forms, including tablets, capsules, suppositories, and liquid.

Nonsteroidal Anti-inflammatory Drugs

Taking NSAIDs (ibuprofen, naproxen, diclofenac, and others) early in pregnancy has been linked to an increased risk for miscarriage. The risk is highest when NSAIDs are used around the time of conception. Using them in the third trimester can also have harmful effects on the baby's heart development, contractions of the uterus, and bleeding. Most doctors in the United States limit NSAIDs to the first and second trimesters, while many European doctors limit their use to only the second trimester because of increased early miscarriage risk. It is safest to restrict NSAIDs to the second trimester only, if they are used at all. Talk to your doctor about whether he or she is comfortable with your use of NSAIDs during your pregnancy.

Aspirin

Aspirin is generally best avoided during pregnancy. Don't be overly concerned if you inadvertently took aspirin in early pregnancy. A review of
research studies and a large population study using information col-
lected through a national registry in Hungary showed no increased risk
of birth defects in babies born to women who used aspirin during the
first trimester. Furthermore, another large study evaluating babies from
over 19,000 pregnancies showed no negative long-term effects on intel-
lectual development in 4-year-olds who were exposed to aspirin during the first 20 weeks of pregnancy.

*Pain-relieving proper-
ties of acetamino-
phen can be boosted
by adding moderate
amounts of caffeine,
which is rated FDA
risk-category B.
Moderate amounts
would be one cup of
coffee or 100 mg of
caffeine.*

Caffeine

Caffeine is a safe therapy that can boost the
pain-relieving effect of analgesic medications.
See Chapter 3 for recommendations on adding
caffeine to acute analgesic therapy. Pregnant
women should avoid excessive caffeine use,
which has undesirable stimulant effects. It's best
to limit use to two cups per day or less of caf-
feinated beverages. Studies do not show any link between using caffeine
during pregnancy and risk for birth defects.

Lidocaine

Lidocaine (LidaMantle®, Xylocaine®) is an FDA category B compound
that is considered safe to use during pregnancy. It will need to be
made into a 4 percent nasal solution for migraine treatment. Not all
pharmacies are able to compound medications in this way, so you may
need to search for a local pharmacy that can make this solution. In a
controlled study, intranasal lidocaine provided short-lived migraine
relief for 1–2 hours in about half of the non-pregnant patients treated.
Controlled studies with pregnant women have not been completed.

To use intranasal lidocaine, lie down and extend your head over the edge of the bed, so that your head tips back. Slowly drip 0.5–1 mL of 4 percent lidocaine (about 10–20 drops) into the nostril on the side of the headache. Repeat 2 minutes later if the headache hasn't gone away. Lidocaine nasal solution is generally well tolerated, but you may notice numbness of the nasal membranes. Topical lidocaine in cream or patch form is also considered safe.

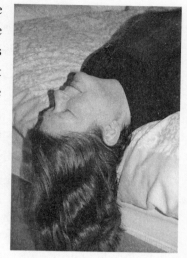

Lying on the bed with your head over the side is a good position when you plan to use intranasal lidocaine.

Migraine-Specific Treatments

Ergotamines are advised to be avoided during pregnancy, including DHE. If you do inadvertently use DHE before you know you're pregnant, don't be alarmed. A study evaluating babies born to over 900 women in Sweden who had used migraine drugs during early pregnancy—most often sumatriptan or an ergotamine—showed no increased birth defects in their babies.

Triptans are among the most effective acute migraine agents. Drug companies continue to collect data in pregnancy registries on women who have used triptans during pregnancy. There is currently no high-quality evidence suggesting an increased risk for birth defects when a triptan was used during pregnancy. Most women who used a triptan during pregnancy used sumatriptan (Imitrex®), and no specific increased risks have been identified.

Don't be overly concerned if you used a triptan during early pregnancy before realizing you were pregnant.

A recent review of available data on sumatriptan treatment concluded that first-trimester treatment of worsening or new-onset migraine is probably safe. Due to the relatively small number of identified women

Triptan Pregnancy Registries

Triptan	Company	Contact
Sumatriptan (Imitrex®)	GlaxoSmith Kline	800-336-2176 in
Naratriptan (Amerge®)		North America
		910-256-0549 outside of North America
Rizatriptan (Maxalt®)	Merck	800-986-8999

who have used triptans during pregnancy, however, strong safety recommendations cannot be confidently made, and these drugs should generally be avoided during pregnancy. If you do take a triptan when you're pregnant, contact the drug company to let them know, so that they can continue to collect data on triptan effects during pregnancy.

Nausea Therapy

Drugs commonly used to treat nausea during pregnancy include the FDA category B drugs metoclopramide (Reglan®), ondansetron (Zofran®), and the FDA category C drug promethazine (Phenergan®). A recent survey found that the nausea medications most commonly prescribed by obstetricians are ondansetron and promethazine. These are available as pills, liquids, dissolvable tablets, and rectal suppository forms.

PREVENTION DRUGS

If you're still experiencing frequent, disabling migraine attacks after the first trimester, you will need to use prevention therapy. If non-medication prevention treatments (such as relaxation therapy and stress management) are not effective, you may need a prevention medication. In general, it's better for you and the baby to take a safe prevention drug than to use excessive analgesic medications or risk poor nutrition and dehydration.

Blood Pressure Drugs

Among headache preventive medications, beta-blockers have the best track record for a combination of effectiveness and safety in pregnant women. Propranolol (Inderal®) is considered the best first-choice prevention drug during pregnancy for most women. Even though it is considered relatively safe, some problems have been noticed with women using blood pressure medications during pregnancy. Beta-blockers, such as propranolol, can increase the baby's risk of having low blood sugar, slow heart rate, low blood pressure, or slowed breathing at birth. Ideally, beta-blockers should be tapered within the last few weeks of pregnancy (starting around week 36) to minimize effects on labor and the newborn baby. Early use of another beta-blocking medication, atenolol (Tenormin®) at conception or during the first trimester has been linked to low birth weight.

Other blood pressure medications, such as the calcium-channel blockers and angiotensin blockers, have been used less extensively in pregnant women. A strong safety record has not yet been established with these drugs, and they should not be used to treat migraines.

Antidepressants

Antidepressants are generally not recommended for headache prevention when you're pregnant, and are generally reserved for the treatment of serious depression during pregnancy. Tricyclic antidepressants such as amitriptyline have been linked to an increased risk of miscarriage and birth defects. Selective serotonin reuptake inhibitors (SSRIs) have been linked to an increased risk for low birth weight and respiratory distress in the newborn. One SSRI drug, paroxetine (Paxil®) has been linked to an increased risk for heart defects in the baby and is now an FDA category D drug. *Bupropion* (Wellbutrin®) has also been linked to an increased risk of miscarriages and heart defects.

Babies exposed to SSRIs and serotonin and norepinephrine reuptake inhibitors have been linked to the development of *behavioral neonatal syndrome.* Babies with this condition may be jittery and irritable, and have problems with feeding, sleeping, and breathing. In most cases, symptoms are mild and do not require specific treatment.

Anti-Seizure Drugs

In general, anti-seizure drugs are limited to the treatment of seizure or epilepsy disorders during pregnancy because studies show a small increase in birth defect risks with this group of medications.

Gabapentin (Neurontin®) may be used in early pregnancy and then discontinued in the third trimester because of possible interference with the baby's bone development. No increased risk for miscarriage, low birth weight, or birth defects have been identified in women using gabapentin during pregnancy. While this is encouraging, gabapentin has not been used in enough pregnancies to know that it is safe to use. If you do take gabapentin when you're pregnant, call the drug company's registry at 617-638-7751. The North American Antiepileptic Drug Pregnancy Registry sponsored by Massachusetts General Hospital is also collecting data on the outcomes of babies exposed to antiepileptic drugs during pregnancy. You can register your information with them by calling 888-233-2334.

Both topiramate (Topamax®) and valproate (Depakene®, Depacon®) have been linked to an increased risk of birth defects. Neither of these antiepileptic drugs should be used for headache prevention during possible conception or pregnancy.

RESCUE THERAPY

Although butalbital medications (such as Fioricet®) can be relatively safe to use during pregnancy, they are not recommended because of their limited effectiveness in treating headache symptoms and the high risk for developing rebound headaches.

Safe Medications During Conception and Pregnancy

	Relatively safe (FDA A or B)	Use if necessary for serious problem (FDA C)
Acute treatments	Acetaminophen (Tylenol®) Caffeine Intranasal lidocaine Nonsteroidal anti-inflammatory drugs during the 2nd trimester (Ibuprofen, naproxen)	Low-dose aspirin Nonsteroidal anti-inflammatory drugs during the 1st trimester Triptans
Nausea medications	Meclizine (Antivert®, Dramamine®) Metoclopramide (Reglan®) Phosphorated carbohydrate solution (Emetrol®) Ondansetron (Zofran®) Doxylamine (Unisom®)	Promethazine (Phenergan®) Prochlorperazine (Compazine®) Chlorpromazine (Thorazine®) Hydroxyzine (Vistaril®)
Prevention therapies	Magnesium	Buproprion (Wellbutrin®) Gabapentin (Neurontin®) Lamotrigine (Lamictal®) Propranolol (Inderal®) Selective serotonin reuptake inhibitor antidepressants (except for paroxetine) Timolol (Blocadren®) Topiramate (Topamax®) Tricyclic antidepressants Venlafaxine (Effexor®) Verapamil (Calan®, Isoptin®)
Rescue drugs	None	Opioids

Opioids (hydrocodone, oxycodone, morphine, and methadone) have a very limited role in migraine and are generally reserved for migraine rescue therapy. Most opioids are FDA risk category C drugs. If you use them, make sure your doctor monitors you carefully. Frequent use of opioids can result in medication overuse headaches. You can also become tolerant to opioids (that is, over time, it takes more medication to get the same effect). You might also experience withdrawal when you stop taking them.

You can also develop a dependency to opioids. Your baby might also develop an opioid dependency from your opioid use and go through withdrawal after birth. Women who have been regularly using daily opioids during mid-to-late pregnancy often need to continue daily opioids for the duration of pregnancy because of the risks to the baby from going through withdrawal *before* birth. It is safer for the baby to experience withdrawal symptoms after birth under the careful supervision of a pediatrician and hospital staff. If you have to use rescue therapy such as opioids, follow these guidelines:

▶ Take your medications only as prescribed.
▶ Only get your pain medications from one provider.
▶ Only get your pain medications from one pharmacy so that there is minimal chance of substitution of one generic source for another.
▶ Don't take other people's pain medications.
▶ Notify your provider if your medications are lost or stolen.

NATURAL REMEDIES FOR MIGRAINE AND NAUSEA

What herbs and supplements can help my migraine symptoms when I'm pregnant?

Several natural remedies are safe for use during pregnancy, but always consult with your physician before adding these preparations to your daily routine. Be sure that your obstetrician and delivery team are aware of any remedies or supplements you are taking.

Acute Treatment

Topical peppermint oil may be safely used during pregnancy.

Nausea Treatment

The American College of Obstetricians and Gynecologists recommends vitamin B6 and ginger for treating pregnancy-related nausea. Controlled clinical trials support the effectiveness and safety of vitamin B6 and ginger for pregnancy-related nausea. In one study, patients were treated with either ginger or vitamin B6 for four days. Nausea severity decreased by about 22 percent with ginger and 17 percent with vitamin B6 after the first day, and by 55 percent with ginger and 31 percent with vitamin B6 after 4 days.

Mild nausea can be treated for up to 3–4 days with ginger 1 gram daily or vitamin B6, 30 mg daily for up to 3–4 days. Both treatments are safe, effective, and recommended by the American College of Obstetricians and Gynecologists.

An-Tai-Yin is another herbal remedy sometimes used to treat morning sickness. It has been linked to an increased risk for birth defects when used during the first trimester. An-Tai-Yin, therefore, should *not* be used during pregnancy or conception.

Prevention Therapy

Magnesium is the only natural remedy recommended as headache prevention during pregnancy; a dose of 400 mg magnesium oxide daily may be used. Safety data are not available for herbs or other supplements during pregnancy, so avoid taking feverfew, butterbur, coenzyme Q10, and high-dose riboflavin.

AFTER PREGNANCY

Whew—I finally delivered! Now what do I do about my headaches?

Congratulations on your new baby! While migraines often disappear or significantly decrease in the second and third trimesters, the majority of women will unfortunately experience an unwelcome return of their headaches after delivery. Also, the stress of learning to care for a new baby and inevitable changes in your sleeping patterns may also trigger additional headaches. Breastfeeding has many benefits—it provides valuable nutrition to your baby, helps you lose that extra "baby fat" that's still hanging on after delivery, and it will help keep your headaches in check.

Fortunately, breastfeeding does offer a protective effect against the return of migraines. Some women are unnecessarily concerned that they'll have to choose between just toughing out migraines with no treatments if they're nursing, or exposing the baby to harmful medications. You shouldn't ignore your headaches after the baby is born. Suffering with untreated, disabling headaches will make it hard for you to enjoy taking care of your baby. The *good* news is that there are a number of effective headache treatments you can use while you're breastfeeding—far more than during pregnancy. You don't have to choose between migraines and nursing. Another piece of good news is that nursing is not expected to aggravate headaches.

Breastfeeding

What Can I Do for My Headaches When I'm Nursing?

These days, after your baby is born, you'll probably only spend a limited amount of time in the hospital and be home for some time before your first visit back to see your doctor. During your final months of pregnancy, be sure to talk to your doctor about a headache treatment plan for after delivery—even if you've stopped having migraines during your pregnancy. You don't want to be caught in the middle of the night with a bad migraine wondering what you can take, if you should just tough it out, or if you should give up your plans for nursing so that you can take the medications you used before becoming pregnant. You will also likely need a prescription for any acute medication that your doctor might recommend for use after delivery. Even if he recommends returning to your previous treatment, you may find that those pills have expired. So before the baby gets here and you're busier than ever, make sure you have an after-delivery treatment plan ready to go.

Before delivery, you will also need to discuss plans for contraception after delivery. Contraception after delivery can be achieved with condoms, spermicides, and/or an intrauterine device. Combined hormonal contraceptives are *not* recommended immediately after delivery, but progestin-only preparations (the "mini pill") may be used. Until you are using reliable contraception, you should follow the same medication restrictions you used when you were pregnant.

Why Is Breastfeeding So Important?

Breastfeeding is terrific for you and your baby! There are numerous health benefits that occur with nursing your baby.

Breastfeeding has important physical and emotional health benefits for you and your baby.

Breastfeeding will:

- ▶ Give your baby optimal nutrition
- ▶ Limit the baby's exposure to foreign proteins
- ▶ Provide necessary hormones, growth factors, and immune complexes
- ▶ Provide important fatty acids to help with good brain development
- ▶ Reduce the risk of infections in the baby
- ▶ Help you and your baby bond with each other

Did you also know that your baby's risk for a variety of medical problems will be significantly lower if you breastfeed? Breastfed babies have significantly reduced risks for developing diarrhea, ear infections, skin disorders, respiratory disease, and even diabetes and leukemia!

Breastfeeding also has substantial perks for *you*! Breastfeeding will:

▶ Help you return to your normal weight

▶ Reduce your risk for breast cancer

▶ Lower your risk for ovarian cancer

▶ Decrease your risk for rheumatoid arthritis

TIPS ON SAFELY PUMPING AND STORING BREAST MILK

▶ Always wash your hands before expressing milk.

▶ Choosing a container for breast milk:

- Use sealable containers, such as bottles with screw tops.

- Wash container with soapy water or clean in the dishwasher before use.

- Use plastic when the milk will be used within a few hours or when refrigerating.

- Use glass when freezing.

- Do not store breast milk in disposable bottle liners.

▶ Amount to put into an individual container:

- Store as 2–4 ounce portions (1/4–1/2 cups).

- You may wish to use a clean ice cube tray for storage—each cube is about 1 ounce. Cover the tray while storing milk.

▶ Acceptable duration of storage for freshly expressed milk:

- Up to 10 hours at room temperature

- Up to 24 hours in cooler with ice packs

- Up to 1 week in refrigerator

  – Store in the back of the refrigerator rather than on door to achieve better maintained temperature.

- Up to 2 weeks in freezer

  – Thaw 12 hours in refrigerator.

  – Never microwave.

  – May refrigerate for 24 hours after thawing.

  – Do not re-freeze.

▶ Delay the return of your migraines during the first month after the baby has been born, and hopefully decrease your headaches

Think of these long-term health benefits as your baby's way of saying "thank you" for your months of pregnancy and hours of delivery!

How Long Should I Plan to Nurse My Baby?

The American Academy of Pediatrics recommends breastfeeding *exclusively* during the first 6 months of a baby's life, with additional nursing recommended for at least the baby's first year. Most mothers nurse during the first few days of a baby's life. Only two of every five mothers are still breastfeeding by the time the baby is 6 months old, and one of every five mothers is nursing when the baby turns 1 year old. There are many reasons why women choose not to breastfeed or to discontinue nursing early. Safety concerns about headache medications and breastfeeding should be carefully reviewed to make sure the decision to nurse or not is based on accurate information.

Acute Treatment During Breastfeeding

You can limit how much medication your baby will get through your breast milk by taking your medicines immediately after completing breastfeeding. This allows the drug you take enough time to be broken down and excreted by your body before your baby's next breastfeeding session. If, on occasion, you need to use acute medications that require cautious use with nursing in order to manage severe migraine attacks, you may wish to pump and store extra breast milk on days when you're not using these drugs. This milk can then be used on days when medication exposure is necessary. If non-compatible drugs are used between feedings, breast milk might be expressed and discarded for several hours after dosing, supplementing feeds with stored milk.

Analgesics During Breastfeeding

Acetaminophen and ibuprofen are the preferred analgesics when breastfeeding. Ibuprofen is generally more effective as a headache rem-

USING MEDICATIONS AFTER DELIVERY AND DURING BREASTFEEDING

Medications that you take when you're nursing may affect your baby, so nursing is another important time to consult your healthcare provider before starting any new treatment. Whether or not your medication will affect the baby depends on a variety of factors:

▶ How much medication makes it into your bloodstream

▶ How much medication gets into the breast milk

▶ How frequently the baby is nursing

▶ How old your breastfeeding baby is

▶ How much medication gets into the baby's bloodstream

▶ What effect each medication might have on the baby

You can make the safest choices for your baby by adjusting the medications you select and how you take those medications:

▶ Select drugs that don't easily get into breast milk.

▶ Choose drugs that are safe for babies to take.

▶ Use the lowest effective dose.

▶ Avoid repeated dosing.

▶ Adjust the time when you take your medication to limit how much will get into your breast milk—and into your baby.

Similar to recommendations during pregnancy, treat mild headaches first with non-drug treatments. Limit medications to more disabling headaches that don't to respond adequately to non-drug therapies.

Breast milk production is quite low for the first 1–2 days after delivery. Medications given during this time are unlikely to be present in your breast milk in concentrations that will likely affect your newborn. After the first few days, when milk production increases, concern about transfer of medications from breast milk to the baby becomes more important.

edy than is acetaminophen. Very little ibuprofen is transferred from the breast milk to the baby. Naproxen is also recommended as safe during breastfeeding by the American Academy of Pediatrics, although naproxen is excreted in small amounts into the breast milk.

Acetaminophen and ibuprofen are the preferred first-line treatment options for headache pain when breastfeeding.

Triptans During Breastfeeding

Sumatriptan was the first triptan developed as acute migraine-specific therapy, and it has been tested in more women than any of the other triptans. Very little sumatriptan is excreted into breast milk. The American Academy of Pediatrics has determined that sumatriptan can be safely used when nursing without needing to pump and discard the milk around the time of feeding. There is not enough information with other triptans to be able to provide safe recommendations for their use when nursing.

Nausea Treatment During Breastfeeding

Information on the safe use of nausea treatments when nursing is limited. The American Academy of Pediatrics has determined that ondansetron is probably safe when nursing. Limited information is available for metoclopramide and prochlorperazine (Compazine®). Promethazine should not be used in children under 2 years old, so caution with nursing may also be needed.

Ondansetron is the preferred treatment for nursing women with nausea.

Prevention Drugs During Breastfeeding

If you're taking a headache prevention therapy, talk to your doctor about using once-daily dosing. You can minimize the amount of drug your baby will get by taking a once-daily medication during the longest time when you won't be nursing, most commonly before your baby's longest period of sleep.

Antidepressants During Breastfeeding
Antidepressants are excreted into breast milk, and the effects of antidepressants on the baby's developing brain and nervous system have not been extensively studied. Therefore, when nursing, antidepressants are typically restricted to the treatment of moderate to severe depression rather than as headache prevention. Tricyclic antidepressants and the antidepressant sertraline (Zoloft®) may be considered for women with frequent, disabling migraines who have failed to improve sufficiently with non-drug treatments.

Blood Pressure Medications During Breastfeeding
Beta-blockers are generally considered to be relatively safe to use when breastfeeding, although the baby should be monitored for slowing of the heart rate, low blood pressure, or breathing problems. Propranolol and timolol (Blocadren®) are preferred beta-blockers for headache prevention when nursing.

Verapamil (Calan®, Verelan®) is also compatible with breastfeeding, although headache prevention is generally more effective with beta-blockers. Information on angiotensin blockers is not available, so these drugs should be avoided.

Antiepileptic Drugs During Breastfeeding
Divalproex sodium (Depakote®) may be used when nursing as long as you are consistently using an effective method of birth control. Remember—divalproex should not be used when trying to get pregnant or during pregnancy, because it has been shown to be *teratogenic*—to produce birth defects. Because of this, it is extremely important to make sure you're consistently using reliable contraception. You should also continue to take a folate supplement if you're using divalproex. Very little divalproex enters breast milk, but your baby should still periodically have her liver and platelet activity checked if you're taking this drug.

Topiramate is excreted into the breast milk, and safety data for the baby are limited. A study of 203 women with epilepsy using topiramate during pregnancy showed an increased risk for cleft palate. Gabapentin is also excreted into the breast milk, although the concentrations in nursing infants are very low. No problems have been reported for babies of nursing mothers using gabapentin; however, because the available information is limited, gabapentin is generally not recommended for headache prevention when nursing.

Rescue Therapy During Breastfeeding

Single doses of opioids can be used cautiously as rescue therapy—repeated dosing should be avoided. Newborns have a limited ability to break down and metabolize opioids such as morphine. Therefore, repeated dosing in mom may result in a build-up of high morphine levels in the newborn. This may cause the baby to have a dangerously low heart rate and problems breathing.

Natural Remedies for Migraine and Nausea During Breastfeeding

What herbs and supplements can help my migraine symptoms when nursing?
    Some natural remedies and supplements are safe to use during breastfeeding. As always, consult with your doctor before adding any of these items to your routine.

Acute Treatment

Topical peppermint oil can be used by women who are nursing—but *not* while you are actually breastfeeding your baby. Peppermint oil should *never* be used near the faces of babies or children, because it can cause potentially dangerous spasms of the breathing system.

Nausea Treatment

Limited data are available about the safety of ginger (such as sipping dilute ginger ale) for treating nausea during breastfeeding, but it is generally considered to probably be safe.

Prevention Therapy

Magnesium and riboflavin may be used as headache prevention when nursing. Safety data are not available for herbs or other supplements, so you should avoid taking feverfew, butterbur, and coenzyme Q10 when breastfeeding.

PUTTING IT ALL TOGETHER

1. Use reliable contraception until you're ready to become pregnant.

2. Make sure your headache pattern is as stable as possible before you try to get pregnant.

3. Talk to your healthcare provider *before* you become pregnant to discuss headache treatment strategy during pregnancy.

4. Master effective non-drug strategies to use with your milder headaches.

5. When you're trying to get pregnant or are pregnant, treat disabling headaches first with acetaminophen. Consider trying nasal lidocaine.

6. Don't forget to treat nausea aggressively with acupressure, vitamin B6, ginger, or ondansetron.

7. Don't take over-the-counter medications or natural products without first discussing them with your doctor. Remember, most of these have not been studied in pregnant women.

8. If you need a prevention treatment when you're pregnant, try propranolol or magnesium first.

9. Breastfeeding is important for you *and* your baby; it helps delay the return of headaches to the pattern you had before pregnancy.

10. When you're nursing, you may use acetaminophen, ibuprofen, and sumatriptan for acute headaches; ondansetron for nausea; and propranolol, timolol, verapamil, magnesium, and riboflavin as prevention therapy. Divalproex may be used if you consistently use an effective contraceptive.

SUMMARY

- ▶ Talk to your healthcare provider about making plans for safe headache treatments during each stage of pregnancy.
- ▶ Learn non-drug treatments before becoming pregnant, so that you are comfortable using them to treat milder headache episodes.
- ▶ Because nausea is often increased during pregnancy, make sure you always have an effective nausea treatment on hand.
- ▶ Remember, it's better to use safe headache medications than to suffer with disabling migraines that might limit your nutritional intake or result in dehydration.
- ▶ Breastfeeding is healthy for you and your baby. Nursing also helps reduce the return of headaches after delivery. You shouldn't expect nursing to make your migraines worse.

7

Tackling Migraines During Menopause

Menopause signals the end of a woman's ability to bear children. It is formally defined as beginning 12 full months after a woman's last menstrual period. During the *perimenopause*—the time leading up to the onset of menopause—periods become more irregular and estrogen levels fluctuate. This time of transition is when a woman's headache pattern may begin to change as well. The transition from perimenopause to menopause—typically lasting anywhere from 2 to 8 years—is often marked by hot flashes, mood swings, vaginal dryness, and other symptoms in addition to changing headache pattern.

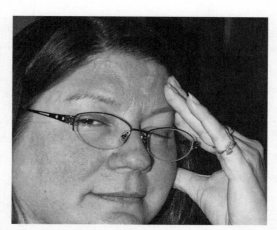

While headaches typically improve in later menopause, women are often unpleasantly surprised when migraines worsen during the early perimenopause.

Hormone replacement therapy (HRT) is sometimes used to treat severe perimenopause symptoms, such as hot flashes and mood swings, and may affect the headache pattern. The good news is that the vast majority of women experience significant improvement and often resolution of their headaches a few years after menopause begins. This is because estrogen levels diminish to very low levels and no longer fluctuate within 2–3 years after menopause begins.

KEY QUESTIONS FOR YOUR DOCTOR

What should I ask about headaches during menopause? I've been having migraine for years. Will these headaches ever end?

Perimenopause and menopause are frequently associated with a change in headache pattern. When perimenopause symptoms begin, you may notice a number of annoying symptoms, including mood swings, hot flashes, vaginal dryness, and a worsening of your headaches. When you are postmenopausal, your headaches usually improve because estrogen levels stop cycling from high to low and stay at a more consistently low level.

COMMON EARLY MENOPAUSE SYMPTOMS

▶ Irregular periods with changes in flow patterns

▶ Vaginal dryness

▶ Hot flashes and night sweats

▶ Disrupted sleep

▶ Mood swings

▶ Increased belly fat

▶ Hair thinning

▶ Decreased sexual drive

▶ Increased headaches

Migraine improves for about two of three women who experience natural menopause. It worsens for about two in three women who have a hysterectomy and removal of the ovaries (surgical menopause).

Any time you experience a significant change in your headache pattern, you should talk to your doctor. What is a *significant* change? See your doctor if:

Talk to your doctor if you develop a new headache pattern or a substantial change in headache activity, or if your usual headache treatments stop working.

- ▶ You develop a new type of headache—even if it's a mild headache
- ▶ Your headaches become much more frequent or more disabling
- ▶ Treatments that usually helped your headaches in the past no longer work
- ▶ You develop new symptoms with your typical headache—such as a new aura
- ▶ You start having other medical problems in addition to your headaches, such as weight loss, fevers, unsteadiness, slurred speech, or extremity weakness

Will Hormone Therapy Affect My Migraines?

Hormone replacement therapy has been routinely used to reduce unpleasant symptoms of early menopause, such as hot flashes, mood swings, and vaginal dryness. In 2002, the Women's Health Initiative study reported that using hormone therapy long-term resulted in more health risks than benefits for some women. This study found slightly increased risks for developing heart disease, breast cancer, stroke, and blood clots in women treated with hormone therapy. The risk was higher in older women who had started menopause more than 10 years before starting HRT. Since that time, doctors have closely examined the results of that study and other studies in women to determine how hormone therapy can be used safely.

RECOMMENDATIONS FOR HORMONE THERAPY DURING MENOPAUSE

Short-term use of hormone therapy can effectively treat menopause symptoms such as hot flashes. This is the primary reason why hormone therapy is used.

▶ Short-term hormone therapy should be considered if you have moderate to severe menopause symptoms that are unresponsive to non-estrogen alternatives.

▶ Hormone replacement may be used in women who are less than 60 years old.

▶ Hormone therapy should be started within 10 years of your first menopause symptoms.

▶ You should be treated with the lowest possible hormone dose to control your symptoms.

▶ If your main symptom is vaginal dryness, consider using a vaginal preparation, to reduce the effects of hormones on the rest of your body.

▶ Use hormone therapy for as short a time period as possible. Talk to your doctor every 6 to 12 months to determine if you should continue hormone therapy.

▶ Short-term use of hormone therapy also prevents bone loss (osteoporosis), but many non-estrogen alternatives are available that work as well or better for osteoporosis and are associated with fewer risks.

▶ Don't use hormone replacement for more than 10 years.

▶ Don't use hormone replacement if you have had breast cancer, heart disease, or blood clots. You should also quit smoking before starting hormone therapy.

▶ If you still have your uterus, you'll need to take progesterone in addition to estrogen.

▶ Get regular annual mammograms while taking hormone therapy.

▶ Consider effective non-hormone therapies such as antidepressants (venlafaxine [Effexor®] and paroxetine [Paxil®]), gabapentin (Neurontin®), and clonidine (Catapres®). Research studies have confirmed that these can be effective agents for perimenopausal symptoms.

RECOMMENDATIONS FOR HORMONE THERAPY DURING MENOPAUSE (CONTINUED)

▶ Include helpful non-drug treatments: relaxation, stress management, yoga, and acupuncture.

▶ Include these lifestyle changes for hot flashes: wear loose fitting clothing, dress in layers, use fans, exercise regularly, avoid hot and spicy foods, and limit caffeine and alcohol.

Using hormone therapy may change your headaches. In general, studies show that hormone therapy has about the same chance of making your headaches better or worse. Unfortunately, the benefit can be difficult to predict. Because hormonal headaches are caused by hormone cycling, you can reduce the effects hormone replacement will have on your headaches by keeping the changes from highest to lowest estrogen levels as small as possible. You can do this by:

▶ Talking to your healthcare provider about using a hormone patch instead of a pill. Using a continuous, transdermal estradiol patch gives you a steadier level of estrogen in your system than taking a pill.

▶ Using the lowest possible hormone dose to control your menopause symptoms.

You may also need to add headache prevention therapy if headaches become a problem when you're using perimenopausal hormones and you need to continue hormones for health reasons. (See Chapter 3 for headache prevention treatments.) You will probably be able to discontinue prevention medications when you stop taking hormone therapy.

Talk to your doctor about what to expect from hormone replacement therapy.

NON-DRUG TREATMENTS

How should I treat migraines during perimenopause and menopause?

The non-drug treatments described in Chapter 3 can be used during perimenopause and menopause.

It's never too late to start using effective non-drug techniques, even for women well past the menopause. Traditionally, doctors thought that seniors would not get much of an effect from pain management skills. However, a research study proved that these skills are also helpful for reducing headaches in seniors, and menopause is a great time to use effective non-drug techniques, even if you haven't used them earlier. Seniors ranging in age from 60 to 77 years old were taught cognitive behavioral therapy, relaxation, and biofeedback. Headaches were reduced by at least half in two of three seniors learning these techniques. Interestingly, women did better than men.

Adopting healthy lifestyle habits may be particularly important during menopause to control headaches and improve overall health.

Non-drug headache treatments such as cognitive behavioral therapy, relaxation, and biofeedback can be effectively learned and used by seniors.

Increased belly fat has been linked to both increased risk for heart disease and an increased risk for hot flashes. A recent study of women in early menopause found that over half gained body fat during the first 3 years of menopause. On average, body fat increased by 2 percent each year. The women who gained body fat were also about 25 percent more likely to experience unpleasant menopause symptoms such as hot flashes. When you are starting menopause, make sure you assess your diet and increase your daily exercise to help keep your weight in check. Don't try skipping meals to reduce calories. Skipping meals commonly triggers headaches, and research shows that women who skip meals tend not to lose weight. Healthy sleep is also linked to improved weight management and headaches, so be sure to include healthy sleeping habits in your daily routine (see Chapter 3).

HEADACHE MEDICATIONS

Will medications help migraines during perimenopause and menopause?

In general, most acute and prevention drugs can be used during the perimenopause and menopause, similar to when you were younger.

With aging, several additional factors need to be considered when selecting drug treatments. First, as you grow older, your body has a decreased ability to metabolize drugs and an increased sensitivity to many side effects. Because of this, your doctor may have you start treatment with the lowest possible doses. In addition, you may have other health problems that can interfere with using headache medications. Make sure you discuss all new health problems with the healthcare providers who prescribe your medications. And, as noted earlier, *never* use someone else's medications—regardless of your age.

Triptans in Seniors

The use of triptans is controversial in seniors because in rare cases these medications have been linked to ischemic heart disease and heart attacks. This concern is primarily limited to older adults and those with known heart artery blockages or definite coronary artery disease. The effects of triptans on the blood vessels that feed the heart were tested in an interesting study in patients with heart disease who were scheduled for an angioplasty procedure to dilate a constricted blood vessel around the heart. During the procedure, they were injected intravenously (IV) with a solution containing either a triptan medication or a comparison placebo. Overall, the diameter of the heart's blood vessel after IV of the triptan was constricted 4–7 percent with the triptan, and 5 percent with the placebo. A few patients had more substantial constrictions, up to 35 percent with the triptan and up to 22 percent with the placebo. This study supports the conclusion that the effects of triptans on heart arteries is relatively small, even in people who already have heart disease. Nevertheless, it is recommended that triptans not be given to anyone who has any significant risk of heart artery blockages or coronary artery disease.

To be safe, most doctors do not use triptans in patients who have heart disease or who have a high risk for heart disease. Heart disease risk factors include:

▶ A history of heart disease, angina, or a heart attack

▶ A history of strokes

▶ Uncontrolled high blood pressure

▶ High cholesterol

▶ Diabetes

▶ Smoking

▶ A family history of early heart disease (male relatives with heart attacks before age 55, female relatives with heart attacks before age 65)

▶ Obesity

▶ Sedentary lifestyle/minimal regular physical activity

You can reduce your risk for heart disease by maintaining a healthy weight, keeping your blood pressure and cholesterol in check, getting checked for diabetes, and quitting smoking. If you are over 60 and still having disabling headaches, talk to your health provider about your heart risk factors and whether you are a candidate to use a triptan medication.

There have also been reports of nonsteroidal anti-inflammatory drugs (NSAIDs) being linked to a slightly higher risk of heart disease events. While this information is preliminary, the small potential risk of NSAIDs must be weighed against their benefit in treating severe headache pain. This may be an more important issue if you already have serious heart disease.

Talk to your doctor about the safety of continuing to use triptans after age 60.

In addition, some women use phosphodiesterase type-5 inhibitors, such as sildenafil (Viagra®), tadalafil (Cialis®), and vardenafil (Levitra®) to enhance the female sexual response, although studies of effects in women have shown inconsistent benefits. If you use these drugs, be aware that headache is a common side effect. Furthermore, the vascular effects of phosphodiesterase type-5 inhibitors oppose those of triptans, so these drugs should generally not be used together.

NATURAL PRODUCTS

Do any natural products help with menopausal headaches?

Vitamins, minerals, and herbs recommended for headache treatment are generally safe and appropriate to use during menopause (see Chapter 3).

Some women opt to treat menopause symptoms with natural estrogen products, called *phytoestrogens*. Phytoestrogens come from plants and are sometimes called *dietary estrogens*. Common sources of phytoestrogens are soy, red clover, and black cohosh. Phytoestrogens have been shown to reduce menopause symptoms, although not all studies show benefit. While phytoestrogens have been shown to reduce menstrual migraines, they have not been specifically tested for migraines after menopause. Studies treating menopausal symptoms with phytoestrogens have shown reductions in headache. Be sure to let your healthcare provider know if you are using phytoestrogens. Although eating dietary

> *Phytoestrogens may reduce menopausal symptoms, including headaches.*

sources of phytoestrogens is likely to be safe, studies have not been conducted to determine if using supplements containing phytoestrogens long-term may have similar health risks to prescription hormone therapy.

PUTTING IT ALL TOGETHER

Menopause is the time when a woman's menstrual cycles stop. The early stages of menopause can be associated with a myriad of symptoms related to estrogen withdrawal, including hot flashes, mood swings, vaginal dryness, and increased headaches. Headaches usually improve in the later stages of menopause, so you may need to increase headache treatments only during perimenopause. General guidelines during this period are:

1. Talk to your doctor about changes in your headache pattern and the effectiveness of your treatments.

2. Maximize your use of non-drug treatments to reduce headaches and other menopause symptoms. Some strategies have been shown to reduce headaches as well as other menopause symptoms. These include stress management, relaxation, cognitive behavioral therapy, sleep hygiene, and exercise.

3. Weight gain is common in early menopause. Minimize weight gain by adopting healthy eating, sleeping, and exercise habits instead of skipping meals.

4. Don't use hormones specifically to treat headaches, because the response is difficult to predict. Talk to your healthcare provider about hormone therapy if you have moderate to severe menopause symptoms, such as hot flashes, vaginal dryness, and mood swings.

5. Use the lowest dose of hormone therapy for the shortest duration possible. If appropriate, consider using vaginal preparations or a transdermal patch instead of pills.

6. You may need to discuss alternatives to triptans if you have a number of risk factors for heart disease.

7. Consider adding prevention therapies if your headaches are frequent.

SUMMARY

▶ Headaches often worsen temporarily during the perimenopause when you are also having other menopause symptoms, such as hot flashes, because of fluctuating estrogen levels.

▶ Hormone replacement therapy is just as likely to make your headaches better or worse, and there are small but definite risks to taking hormone therapy.

▶ If you need to use hormone replacement for perimenopausal symptoms, talk to your doctor about trying vaginal therapy or a patch.

▶ Most non-drug treatment options, medications, and natural products that are generally effective for headache treatment will continue to be effective during menopause.

8

Learning How to Talk
to Your Healthcare Provider

Have you ever had trouble talking to your doctor? Do you sometimes feel like he's not really hearing what you're saying, or not answering your questions? If you often feel like this, you're probably leaving your doctor's office frustrated and confused. By using simple strategies, you should be able to improve how well you and your healthcare provider communicate.

Talking to your healthcare provider can be difficult, and many things can make the visit less than satisfying. Some doctors seem unapproachable or aloof. Sometimes there are too many things to cover in the time allotted. Some seem too busy to answer your questions. This type of problem can make it difficult for you to have your concerns heard. It is important to use your time in the office efficiently. Remember that you and your doctor have similar goals in mind—both of you want to help improve your headache pattern.

Open communication and dialogue is the beginning of good headache treatment. Both doctors and patients often fail to express their thoughts and concerns clearly. Doctors may not completely explain your diagnosis and treatment recommendations, and you may be reluctant to openly verbalize your fears and concerns. It may be difficult for you to let your doctor know you're not sure how to use your

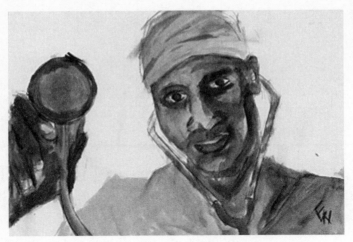

Learning effective communication skills can make your doctor seem more approachable.

prescribed treatment. When this happens, even the best headache recommendations may fail to produce the intended results.

Check out the dialogue here between a doctor and headache patient. The column on the left shows what each actually said. The right column shows what they were trying to say. You'll notice that both the patient and her doctor did a poor job of getting their messages across. Read through the dialogue and see if you can recognize yourself or your doctor. As is often the case, the exchange of useful information is poor because both the doctor and patient are not being as clear as they could be.

Poor communication in the doctor's office is unfortunately very common. In the American Migraine Communication Study, migraine patient visits to healthcare providers were videotaped and later analyzed by researchers. The average visit lasted only 12 minutes. During visits, patients were most often asked about migraine frequency. Doctors rarely asked about how migraines impacted people's daily lives. Perhaps most importantly, over half of the doctors and their patients disagreed on how often the patients had migraines and the level of impairment people experienced with their migraines. This study emphasized what

A TYPICAL MIGRAINE OFFICE VISIT

What they actually said	What they wanted to communicate
Doctor: Tell me about your headaches, Ms. Jenkins.	I hope she gets right to the point. I'm already 20 minutes behind schedule!
Patient: Well, I first started getting bad migraines when I was 12 years old.	I brought 10 years worth of reports for him to review, and he never even looked at them!
Doctor: Yes, yes, that's fine. How frequent are your headaches now?	Doesn't she realize I've already read 10 years worth of records about her? Why did she bring all of these if she's going to tell me every detail that's in them anyway!
Doctor: I see you brought your brain scan. Let me show it to you. Here's your brain, and this is the skull. And see these little white spots? They're high-signal intensity abnormalities on T2-weighted images that can occur with headache.	This is a normal brain scan. There is no tumor or abnormal blood vessels. About one in every three people with migraines will have these small white spots. These spots are nothing to worry about and are not a sign of any disease or damage.
Patient: Oh.	Does he think I have a brain tumor?
Doctor: Migraine is caused by chemical imbalances in the brain. Serotonin imbalance causes the blood vessels around the brain to react abnormally and this causes headache.	Migraine is not serious. There is no reason to worry.
Patient: So will I need surgery? Is it serious? Is it fatal?	Abnormal blood vessels! My uncle died of a brain aneurysm—is that what I've got? What's serotonin, and how did I get it?
Doctor: You don't have any serious problem, and you don't need surgery. Are you depressed?	She's not even listening to me! She seems very keyed up and anxious. Maybe she has a mood disorder—not

FEATURES OF THE AVERAGE MIGRAINE (CONTINUED)

What they actually said	What they wanted to communicate
	unusual with chronic headache. Maybe that's why she's not focusing on what I'm telling her. Luckily some migraine medications treat both.
Patient (with tears welling up in her eyes): Not at all!	Not again! Everyone thinks I'm making up my headaches! Why doesn't my doctor take my migraines seriously?!
Doctor: For people with your particular condition, we often use antidepressants. And we'll have you meet with the psychologist. They have good treatments for you. Biofeedback and relaxation are also effective migraine therapies.	She's in denial. Maybe this mood problem is more serious than I thought! Antidepressants are great headache preventive medications, so that would be a good choice.
Patient: How do I take these?	He really does think I'm just crazy. I'll try these pills and see if they help. I'm so desperate at this point I'd try anything!
Doctor: Just take one pill before you go to bed, and I'll see you back in 4 weeks.	She needs to take this every day for several weeks before it will work.
Patient: Okay. Before you go, I wanted to ask a few questions. Here's a list I wrote down for you.	I wonder what the side effects are. I'll take it a couple of times and see if it works.
Doctor: Here are a couple of pamphlets. We'll answer any remaining questions at your next visit.	She brought four pages of questions! I don't have time to answer four pages worth of questions today.
Four weeks later...	
Doctor: Feeling better, Ms. Jenkins? You're taking that pill I gave you every day, right?	She's not complaining so the headaches must have improved.

FEATURES OF THE AVERAGE MIGRAINE (CONTINUED)

What they actually said	What they wanted to communicate
Patient: Uh, no. I just take it when I have a bad headache before I go to sleep like you said.	It's not working at all! But if I complain you'll dismiss me as a patient and then what will I do?
Doctor: I'll have my nurse come talk to you. Good-bye for now, Ms. Jenkins.	Oh, good grief! I specifically told her to take it every day! Maybe my nurse will get the medication instructions straight. I'll see her again in a couple of more weeks to check on things.
Patient: Good-bye, doctor.	That's it. I'm being dismissed by the nurse. He won't even speak to me. Time to find a new doctor.

---

many already suspected—communication in the exam room is often far less than ideal.

The good news is that you *can* improve communications with your healthcare provider—even if your healthcare provider is not a very

---

IS POOR COMMUNICATION AFFECTING HEADACHE VISITS?

When you're with your healthcare provider, do you find yourself thinking:

1. My doctor never seems to understand what I'm saying.

2. My doctor's directions are always vague and unclear.

3. I never get to ask the questions that are really important to me.

4. Talking to my doctor is like talking to a wall.

5. My doctor has the bedside manner of a rock.

6. My doctor has no idea how my life is affected by my headaches.

If you typically find yourself leaving your doctor's office frustrated and having these kinds of thoughts, you need to work on developing better communication with your healthcare provider.

good communicator. By using effective communication strategies yourself, you can significantly improve the value of your office visit. Modeling effective communication techniques, such as those listed here, may also help your healthcare provider learn how to improve communications with you and other patients! Taking time to effectively communicate makes the visit more productive and satisfying.

FOCUS ON THE MOST IMPORTANT QUESTIONS

Knowing What to Ask

When you are initially seen for your headaches, you will likely have many questions about your headache condition. Since there is a lot to cover and time is limited, make sure you use this time wisely. Prioritize your questions and get the most important ones answered first.

You'll probably get the best results if you limit yourself to asking three or four major questions at each visit. Don't expect to get everything addressed during one visit. Save these less pressing questions to ask at a later visit.

You will also get the most useful answers if you ask direct questions. For example, if your doctor wants you to take an antidepressant for your headaches, don't be afraid to say, "I don't think I'm depressed. I'm just very frustrated with these headaches, and I'm afraid no one believes that anything is wrong. Do you think I have a mental disorder?" Doctors have a much easier time answering pointed questions. In this particular case, the patient should understand that doctors use certain antidepressant medications at times because they affect certain brain chemicals that are important not only in depression, but also for chronic pain. By clarifying this, it is easier to understand why the doctor is prescribing the medication.

MAKE CERTAIN YOU UNDERSTAND
YOUR DIAGNOSIS

Understanding Why You're Getting Headaches

Don't leave your visit without finding out what your doctor thinks is causing your headaches. Ask your doctor directly, "What's causing my headaches?" Realize that you may not get a definitive answer at the first visit. If the doctor can't give you a headache diagnosis, that doesn't necessarily mean that the headaches are caused by something serious. Modern medicine does a good job figuring out what problems you *don't* have. You don't have a brain tumor. You don't have an aneurysm. It's often more difficult to figure out what you *do* have. Your doctor should be able to at least give you a general idea about what is likely to be the reason for your headaches, even before a definite diagnosis has been reached.

Headaches are diagnosed by matching your headache description to typical headache patterns. When your headache pattern is not typical, this can be more difficult. The doctor may need to review old tests you had done, order new tests, or confer with a colleague. Reviewing several weeks or months of headache diaries may also help determine your headache diagnosis. It is most time-efficient if you review your pattern before the visit and be ready to summarize it. For example, you may report that you tend to have on average 5–7 headaches per month with at least half of them consistently beginning 1–2 days before your menstrual period begins. Or, you might tell the doctor that your

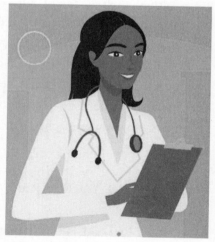

Make sure you understand what your doctor thinks is causing your headaches before leaving your appointment.

headaches seemed to get worse about 3 weeks ago after you started your new job. Observations such as these, based on your headache diary, can help direct treatment decisions.

SHARE YOUR CONCERNS AND REACTIONS

Tell Your Healthcare Provider What Is Really Worrying You

If there's something that you're especially worried about, be sure to ask about it directly. For example, you may ask, "Do you think my headaches are caused by a brain tumor?" or "Can this medication affect my mood? Ever since I started that new prevention medication, I've been blue and weepy." If you don't bring these types of things up, your doctor may assume that they are not present and move on.

A good way to make sure that you understand what your healthcare provider tells you is to rephrase what you're hearing to be certain you have it right. Ask questions such as, "So you're saying my headaches are inherited migraines and not caused by something serious like a brain tumor or infection, right?" And, "When you say to take this pill every day for my headache, do you mean that I need to take it every single day whether I have a headache or not, *or* do you only want me to take it on the days when I have a headache?" These questions will help clarify what your doctor is telling you and what you need to do to help get relief from your headache pain.

UNDERSTAND YOUR TREATMENT RECOMMENDATIONS

Know How to Treat Your Headaches

Headache treatment can be complicated. Writing down the instructions and reviewing them before you leave the office will make it easier to remember how to treat your headaches at home. Acute-care medicines cannot be taken more than a few days per week, while preventive medicines must be used daily in order to work. It also may take 2–3 months to get the full benefit of preventive medications. While some doctors will review the headache treatment plan with you, others may have their nurse or assistant explain the headache program to you. It is a good idea to carefully write down your headache treatment program and confirm that this is the correct strategy. Also, you can ask your pharmacist to clarify any medication questions that weren't asked or answered in the doctor's office. It is *essential* that you have a good idea of how and when to take your medications and what they are for.

What to Do Before Your Visit

Prepare for your doctor's visit by gathering information about your headaches. Try to organize information describing your headache pattern and figure out what questions you need to have answered right away. Here are some hints to help you get started:

▶ *Keep a headache diary for 1–2 months before your visit*, if possible, and bring it to the visit. See Chapter 3 for a sample diary you might use.

▶ *Try to summarize your past treatments for headache*, noting what worked, what didn't, and which medications weren't tolerated well.

▶ *Collect all of your current medications* and be ready to bring them to the visit.

▶ *Get any old records that pertain to your past headache treatment*, including the results of tests. You do not generally need to bring in the actual X-rays unless the doctor specifically asks to review them. Don't expect the doctor to review them during the office visit. Often she will review them after you leave if there are questions about your history.

▶ *Write down a list of questions that you want answered.* Prioritize them by selecting three or four that are the most important for you to have answered right away.

▶ *Visit one or more of the websites about headaches* listed later in the next chapter to get a general understanding about headaches.

▶ *Sometimes it is helpful to bring in a friend or relative with you who can act as an extra pair of ears regarding the instructions and explanations.*

Preparing for your visit in advance is the best way to make sure that your healthcare provider will have what she needs to best determine what's causing your headaches and what treatments are most likely to be helpful.

What to Talk About at Your First Headache Visit

Make Certain You Share Essential Information

Make sure you give your doctor complete information about your migraines and any other health problems. Migraine symptoms you need to tell your doctor about include:

▶ How often you get a migraine

▶ How long your migraines usually last

▶ How disabling your migraines are—for example, do you miss work or school because of your headaches, or do you miss going to family functions or social activities because of headaches, or because you're afraid you might get a headache?

▶ What treatments you have tried in the past

▶ Whether you also get other headaches regularly

Make sure you tell your doctor about:

- ▶ Other medical conditions that you're being treated for
- ▶ Any history of head or neck trauma or surgery
- ▶ All of the pills you take and their dosages—including over-the-counter and natural remedies. It's best to bring in all of your medications for every visit to make sure your doctor knows exactly what you're taking.
- ▶ Any other treatment you're getting
- ▶ Plans for conception and possible pregnancy

QUESTIONS YOU SHOULD ASK AT EVERY VISIT

Make Sure You Understand Your Headaches and How to Treat Them

When you leave each appointment, make sure you can answer all of these questions:

- ▶ What is my headache diagnosis?
- ▶ How should I take my medication?
- ▶ How long should this medicine take to work?
- ▶ What main side effects should I watch for?
- ▶ When should I make my next visit?

Don't be afraid to ask why a specific treatment was prescribed. Migraine sufferers often wonder in silence why their doctors prescribed certain treatments. This can be compounded when they go home and the family says, "Your doctor doesn't know what he's doing! He gave you a blood pressure pill instead of a headache pill!" or "We told you it was all in your head and you were just depressed." When you don't understand why a treatment is prescribed, it may be more difficult for you to be compliant with the medication and take it every day. It is always preferable for you as a patient to be interested and directly involved in your care. Your doctor should be able to clearly explain why a specific treatment was prescribed. Don't be afraid to say you don't understand why something was prescribed for you.

Be sure to regularly talk to your healthcare provider about hormonal relationships you've noticed with your headaches and about plans to start or add to your family. Also, let your doctor know any preferences you have for non-drug or natural therapies, and talk about including these treatments in a medication regimen during different life stages.

SUMMARY

▶ Make sure you develop good communication skills with your healthcare provider.

TIPS FOR SUCCESSFUL COMMUNICATION

▶ Prepare for every visit with your healthcare provider. Write down and bring a list of concerns—prioritize those key concerns that are most important for you.

▶ Ask specific questions that are of most concern to you right now and save less-urgent questions for a later visit.

▶ Use direct and specific questions, such as how long should I wait to take the next acute medication.

▶ Restate what you hear your doctor saying to make sure you understand. For example, "so, let me get this straight—you think that my headaches are migraines without aura and you want me to take this medication Topamax every night to reduce headache frequency—right?"

▶ Speak up about any concerns that you have about your diagnosis, treatment, or other symptoms.

▶ Keep your doctor informed about hormonal links with your headache, your current method of contraception, plans for conceiving, concerns about pregnancy, and changes with menopause.

▶ Do your homework. There are many excellent books and websites about headaches (see Chapter 9). Knowledge is power!

▶ Be prepared for each headache visit. Write questions down, prioritize them, bring your headache diary with you (and summarize the pattern if possible). Bring all of your medications to every visit.

▶ Don't get discouraged if you can't get all of your questions answered right away. Learn to prioritize what you need to know.

▶ Learn as much as you can about headaches—the more you know, the more you will feel that you are in control of your headaches.

9

Resource Guide

Where Can I Get More Information?

K*nowledge is power.* Research consistently shows that educating yourself about your headaches helps you get them under better control. The more you know, the more you will feel in control of your headaches. In one study, migraine sufferers were given written information about headaches, including information about common headache triggers, healthy lifestyle recommendations, and instructions about how to learn relaxation techniques and stress management. Materials were sent by mail, so the benefits occurred from self-education rather than from additional interventions from healthcare providers. After 8 weeks, headaches were substantially improved:

- Headache frequency dropped by 37 percent.
- Headache disability decreased by 71 percent.
- Depression symptoms decreased by 29 percent.
- Migraine sufferers' confidence that they could effectively manage their headaches improved by 22 percent.

Your healthcare provider can also be an excellent resource for headache information, as well as answering questions about diagnosis and treatment options. There are also many reliable sources of informa-

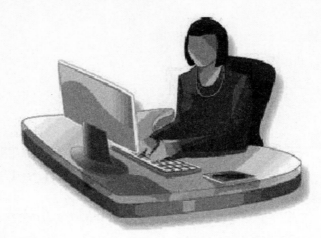

Get Internet information from sites developed by recognized headache authorities for the most accurate and up-to-date information.

tion about headaches, including Internet sites and books written by headache experts. Your healthcare provider can help you sift through the huge amount of information available on headaches, separating the information that is accurate and useful from the information that is not. Together, you can use this information to better understand your condition and develop an effective treatment strategy.

FINDING RELIABLE INTERNET RESOURCES

Some of the best sites for getting reliable and up-to-date headache information are managed by national headache and pain foundations and recognized migraine experts:

- ▶ American Council for Headache Education at http://www.achenet.org
- ▶ American Headache Society at http://www.americanheadachesociety.org
- ▶ National Headache Foundation at http://www.headaches.org

- ▶ National Pain Foundation at
  http://www.nationalpainfoundation.org
- ▶ Help for Headaches & Migraine at
  http://www.helpforheadaches.com
- ▶ Migraine Awareness Group at http://www.migraines.org/about
- ▶ My Migraine Connection at
  http://www.healthcentral.com/migraine
- ▶ Migraine Survival at http://www.migrainesurvival.com

These sites provide information on headache testing, diaries, diets, and treatment, as well as results of new headache research studies.

iHeadache is a headache tracking program that you can use on your iPhone, iPod Touch, and Blackberry. You can find out more at www.iHeadacheApp.com.

You might also enjoy listening to a weekly podcast of migraine information by writer and nationally known headache patient advocate Teri Roberts at http://www.migrainecast.com.

Menstrual Migraine

- ▶ http://www.menstrualmigraine.org
- ▶ http://www.relieve-migraine-headache.com
  menstrual-migraine.html
- ▶ http://www.nationalpainfoundation.org/articles/708/
  menstrual-migraine

Medications During Pregnancy and Breastfeeding

- ▶ The Hospital for Sick Children of the University of Toronto at
  http://www.motherisk.org
- ▶ King's College London at http://www.safefetus.com

- Thomas W. Hale, RPh, PhD, Professor of Pediatrics at Texas Tech University at http://neonatal.ttuhsc.edu/lact
- www.americanpregnancy.org

Tips on Successful Breastfeeding

- http://www.llli.org [La Leche League International website]
- http://www.breastfeed-essentials.com/storagehandling.html
- http://www.breastfeedingbasics.com

Headaches in Children

- http://kidshealth.org
- http://www.migraineadventure.org.uk
- http://www.headaches.org/education/NHF_HeadLines_Excerpts/ Kids_Korner_Archive

Menopause Headaches

- http://www.relieve-migraine-headache.com menopause-headache.html
- http://www.34-menopause-symptoms.com
- http://www.everydayhealth.com/menopause/managing-hormones-and-headaches.aspx
- http://www.menopause.org [North American Menopause Society]

Smoking

- Call 1-800-QUIT-NOW or visit http://1800quitnow.cancer.gov, a website developed by the United States Department of Health and Human Services, National Institute of Health, and National Cancer Institute.

Biofeedback

▶ An inexpensive finger thermometer and biofeedback audiotape can be obtained from Primary Care Network (1-800-769-7565).

Acupressure

▶ Thera Cane® (http://www.theracane.com), a curved cane with knobs placed to help you get to hard-to-reach trigger points.

Mouth Splint

▶ Nociceptive Trigeminal Inhibition (NTI) mouth splint for the prevention of migraine; see www.nti-tss.com.

Nutritional Project and Supplements

▶ Butterbur: www.migraineaid.com
▶ Higher-dose feverfew manufactured in Israel is available from Galilee Herbal Remedies: http://www.relieve-migraine-headache.com/feverfew-migraine.html.

READ A GOOD BOOK

Many excellent books describe effective ways of managing your headaches. Be sure to check out the credentials of the books' authors to help determine if the information is likely to be accurate and reliable. Avoid publications that focus on a single treatment and those that are designed to promote specific products.

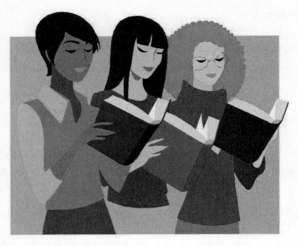

Learning new headache information can help you stay up-to-date with your migraine treatments.

General Information

▶ *The Migraine Brain: Your Breakthrough Guide to Fewer Headaches, Better Health.* Written by neurologist Dr. Bernstein and Elaine McArdle. Published in 2008 by Free Press.

▶ *Managing Migraine: A Patient's Guide to Successful Migraine Care.* Written by family practitioner and headache specialist Dr. Roger Cady and colleagues. Published in 2008 by Baxter Publishing.

▶ *Migraine: Your Questions Answered.* Written by C. A. Foster. Published in 2007 by DK Publishing.

▶ *Living Well with Migraine Disease and Headaches: What Your Doctor Doesn't Tell You … That You Need to Know.* Written by headache expert and patient advocate Teri Roberts. Published in 2005 by Harper Collins.

▶ *Migraines Be Gone: 7 Simple Steps to Eliminating Your Migraines Forever.* Written by educator Kelsie Kenefick. Published in 2006 by Roots and Wings Publishing.

▶ *10 Simple Solutions to Migraine.* Written by neurologist Dr. Dawn Marcus. Published in 2006 by New Harbinger.

Menstrual Migraine

▶ *Menstrual Migraine.* Written by family practitioner and headache expert Susan Hutchison. Published in 2008 by Oxford University Press.

Pregnancy and Breastfeeding

▶ *How to Relieve Headaches During Pregnancy.* Written by headache experts. Published in 2008 by Quick Easy Guides.

▶ *Breastfeeding: Lifesaving Techniques and Advice for Every Stage of Nursing.* Written by educator Suzanne Fredregill. Published in 2007 by Adams Media.

▶ *Drugs in Pregnancy and Lactation: A Reference Guide to Fetal and Neonatal Risk, 8th edition.* Written by obstetrician Dr. Griggs and colleagues. Published in 2008 by Lippincott Williams & Wilkins. This book is a bit technical and may be most helpful if you have a medical background.

▶ *Medications and Mothers' Milk: A Manual of Lactational Pharmacology.* Written by pharmacist Thomas Hale. Published in 2008 by Pharmasoft Medical Publishing.

▶ *The ABCs of Breastfeeding: Everything a Mom Needs to Know for a Happy Nursing Experience.* Written by nurse Stacey Rubin SH. Published in 2008 by AMACOM.

Menopause

▶ *The Menopause Book.* Written by Pat Wingert and Barbara Kantrowitz. Published in 2009 by Workman Publishing.

▶ *The No-Nonsense Guide to Menopause.* Written by Barbara Seaman and Laura Eldridge. Published in 2009 by Simon & Schuster.

▶ *The Cleveland Clinic Guide to Menopause.* Written by internist Dr. Thacker. Published in 2009 by Kaplan Publishing.

▶ *Menopause Sucks: What to Do When Hot Flashes and Hormones Make You and Everyone Else Miserable.* Written Joanne Kimes and Elaine Ambrose. Published in 2008 by Adams Media.

Guides to Learning Non-Drug Treatments

Relaxation and Stress Management

▶ *The Mindfulness Solution to Pain.* Written by psychologist Jackie Gardner-Nix. Published in 2009 by New Harbinger.

▶ *The Relaxation & Stress Reduction Workbook.* Written by psychologist Martha Davis. Published in 2008 by New Harbinger.

▶ *Biofeedback. You Are in Control. Feel. Think. Act!* Written by psychologist Yigal Gliksman. Published in 2008 by Lulu.com.

▶ *Headache Relief (Guided Self-Healing Practices).* Written by physician and acupuncturist Dr. Rossman. Published in 2006 by Sounds True [Audio CD].

▶ *Mindfulness for Beginners.* Written by psychologist Jon Kabat-Zinn. Published in 2006 by Sounds True [Audio CD].

Exercise

▶ *Trigger Point Therapy for Headaches & Migraines.* Written by acupuncturist and neuromuscular therapist Valerie DeLaune. Published in 2008 by New Harbinger.

▶ *Yoga Therapy for Headache Relief.* Written by family practitioner Dr. Van Houten. Published in 2003 by Crystal Clarity Publishers.

Sleep

▶ *Say Good Night to Insomnia.* Written by Harvard professor and behaviorist Gregg Jacobs. Published in 2009 by Holt Paperbacks.

▶ *The Harvard Medical School Guide to a Good Night's Sleep.* Written by sleep specialist Dr. Epstein. Published in 2006 by McGraw-Hill.

Diet

▶ *Tell Me What to Eat If I Have Headaches and Migraine.* Written by dietician Elaine Magee. Published in 2008 by Career Press.

▶ *The Migraine Cookbook: More Than 100 Healthy and Delicious Recipes for Migraine Sufferers.* Written by director of The Migraine Association of Canada, Michele Sharp. Published in 2002 by Marlowe & Co.

Helping Your Child with Headaches

▶ *The Relaxation & Stress Reduction Workbook for Kids.* Written by psychologist Lawrence Shapiro. Published in 2009 by New Harbinger.

▶ *Headache in Children and Adolescents.* Written by pediatric neurologists Drs. Winner and Rothner. Published in 2007 by PMPH.

▶ *Be the Boss of Your Pain: Self-Care for Kids.* Written by pediatrician Dr. Culbert and certified pediatric nurse practitioner Rebecca Kajander. Published in 2007 by Free Spirit Publishing.

▶ *The Headache Detective: Mom, My Head Hurts.* Written by the dad of a child with headaches, John Ricker. Published in 2006 by Thomas and Clayton Publishing.

▶ *Relieve Your Child's Chronic Pain: A Doctor's Program for Easing Headaches, Abdominal Pain, Fibromyalgia, Juvenile Rheumatoid Arthritis, and More.* Written by pediatric pain specialist Dr. Krane. Published in 2005 by Fireside.

▶ *Conquering Your Child's Chronic Pain: A Pediatrician's Guide for Reclaiming a Normal Childhood.* Written by pediatrician Dr. Zeltzer and Christina Blackett Schlank. Published in 2005 by HarperCollins.

Herbal Therapies

▶ *Clinical Botanical Medicine: Revised & Expanded.* Written by naturopath Eric Yarnell and colleagues. Published in 2009 by Mary Ann Liebert.

▶ *The ABC Clinical Guide to Herbs.* Edited by founder of the American Botanical Council Mark Blumenthal. Published in 2003 by Thieme.

▶ *The Nursing Mother's Herbal.* Written by botanist Sheila Humphrey. Published in 2003 by Fairview Press.

Index

Note: Boldface numbers indicate illustrations; *t* indicates a shaded box or table.